Simon Andreae is a journalist and television producer whose series have ranged over the nature of the American presidency, the global history of food, and the science of sexual desire. Often controversial but always entertaining, his films about sexuality include 'The Clitoris Uncovered', 'Geisha', 'Animal Passions', 'Beyond Love' and the series *Anatomy of Desire*, which was based on this book.

He was born in 1966, graduated from Edinburgh University in 1989, and now lives in London with his wife and family. This is his first book.

THE SECRETS
OF LOVE
AND LUST

SIMON ANDREAE

An *Abacus* Book

First published in Great Britain in 1998 as
Anatomy of Desire: The Science and Psychology of Sex, Love and Marriage
by Little, Brown and Company
This edition published in 2000 by Abacus

A CIP catalogue record for this book
is available from the British Library.

ISBN: 0 349 11144 8

Typeset in Berkeley by
Palimpsest Book Production Limited,
Polmont, Stirlingshire
Printed and bound in Great Britain by
Clays Ltd, St Ives plc

Abacus
A Division of
Little, Brown and Company (UK)
Brettenham House
Lancaster Place
London WC2E 7EN

For Lisa

Contents

List of Illustrations

Section One: Basic Instincts

John Adams, the last surviving *Bounty* mutineer on the island of Pitcairn. Of the fourteen others, one died of natural causes, one committed suicide, and twelve were murdered in their struggle for the few available women. (HULTON GETTY)

A light micrograph of DNA (deoxyribonucleic acid). It was strands like these, grouped together and hidden within a protective membrane of fats, which led to the evolution of all life-forms. (PHILIPPE PLAILLY/SCIENCE PHOTO LIBRARY)

The Harem by Thomas Rowlandson. Wherever there have been resources to acquire and land to dominate, men have fought fiercely for supremacy, then directed their energies towards accumulating and enjoying the maximum number of women. (BRITISH MUSEUM)

The pontiff as holy man: Pope Alexander VI, better known by his birth-name Rodrigo Borgia, from the fresco by Pinturicchio in the Borgia apartments of the Vatican. (HULTON GETTY)

The pontiff as beast: Borgia took twenty-five prostitutes into his quarters most nights, and arranged the infamous 'Joust of Whores', in which naked women were obliged to race on all fours down paths illuminated by candles, while Borgia and his friends attempted to mount whichever took their fancy. (TOPHAM)

Illustration inspired by Vatsyayana's *Kama Sutra*. From the Pacific atolls to the Amazon jungles, from the wastelands of Waco to the royal palaces of Brunei, men have seen women as the currency, the incentive, and the reward of power. (PRIVATE COLLECTION)

Matt and Eric, F-to-Ms from Seattle, Washington. (DEL LAGRACE VOLCANO)

A cross-section of the human brain showing Paul MacLean's 'triune' hierarchy: brain stem, limbic system and cortex. (DAVID GIFFORD/SCIENCE PHOTO LIBRARY)

A sketch of Juliane Lipka, one of the murderesses of Nagyrev. Over one hundred men were killed in the village between 1914 and 1929 after their spouses had experienced real sexual freedom for the first time.

Husband-and-wife team William Masters and Virginia Johnson, who collaborated on a detailed examination of female sexuality whose results were published in their book *Human Sexual Response*. (CORBIS-BETTMANN/UPI)

The University of Amsterdam's Sex Chair, which uses an array of instruments to measure the sexual responses – both conscious and unconscious – of whoever sits in it. (OPTOMEN TV)

The guarantee of satisfaction: Rita Clay Estrada's *The Stormchaser*, one of a series of highly successful romantic novels in which the hero always promises his long-term and exclusive care – a principal factor in female desire. (HARLEQUIN MILLS & BOON)

One of the best-selling images of the 1980s. Pictures of model Adam Perry on his own sold steadily, but once he got hold of the baby, sales rocketed. (SPENCER ROWELL PRODUCTIONS)

A female club-goer in Vienna being examined by Professor Karl Grammer. In a series of experiments Grammer found that women were most likely to be unfaithful on the very nights when they were most likely to conceive. (OPTOMEN TV)

'Madonna' . . . (ARMANDO GALLO/RETNA)

. . . or 'whore'? Actually, depending on their mood, the time of the month, the men presented to them, and any number of other factors, most women could be both. (NEAL PRESTON/RETNA)

Section Two: Shaping Forces

The Venus of Willendorf: matriarchal goddess, Stone Age centrefold or 30,000-year-old fertility symbol? (ALI MEYER/BRIDGEMAN ART LIBRARY)

Sketch showing the 'Red Threesome', the Ice Age remains of two men and a woman found in a shallow grave in the Czech Republic. Is this the first formal record of humanity's violent sanctions against adultery? (COURTESY OF TIMOTHY TAYLOR)

A five-year-old Indian bride watches her fifteen-year-old husband during their wedding ritual. In Rajasthan in August 1985, 50,000 children were promised to each other in a series of mass betrothals over two days. (POPPERFOTO)

Marriage, Western-style: a traditional British white wedding. (EMMA LEE/LIFE FILE)

From the eleventh century, many Chinese women had their feet bound. Soon the results of the binding became a fetish in themselves. (POPPERFOTO)

Afghan women living under the extreme Islamic code of the Taliban. Heavy veiling such as this sends a clear signal that these women are taken, and not available to any men other than their husbands. (POPPERFOTO)

'The wages of sin is death.' Punishment by stoning, as portrayed by Gina Lollobrigida in King Vidor's *Solomon and Sheba*. (THE KOBAL COLLECTION)

Marshall Applewhite, leader of the Heaven's Gate cult in California, seen here in a still from the videotape made shortly before he and thirty-eight others committed suicide. (POPPERFOTO)

The Conversion of St Paul by Alonso Berruguete. Paul's famous letters to the Corinthians have formed the bedrock of Christian thinking on matters of sex and marriage ever since. (E. T. ARCHIVE)

St Augustine by El Greco. According to Augustine, lust was not a natural part of creation but a disease introduced into human nature at the moment of the Fall, responsible for the expulsion from Eden and staining every generation from that day to this. (E. T. ARCHIVE)

The Assumption of the Virgin by Titian. Following on from the teachings of Paul, Jerome and Augustine on the virtues of virginity, it became all the more essential to emphasise that Jesus himself had been born untainted by sin. His mother's virginity, therefore, soon grew from an apocryphal folk-tale to a central pillar of the Christian faith. (E. T. ARCHIVE)

'Day and night, long processions of all classes and ages, headed by priests carrying crosses and banners, perambulated the streets in double file, praying and flagellating themselves.' By the mid-thirteenth century, self-flagellation had become a popular penance throughout Europe. (MARY EVANS PICTURE LIBRARY)

The S/M scene today often draws heavily on Christian iconography and fetishes: the cross, the confessional, the miserable sinner and the unforgiving God. (HOUSK RANDALL)

The book that started all the trouble: frontispiece for an early edition of *Onania*, which railed in the most colourful terms about the evils of masturbation, with one of the alleged results, according to a Victorian health manual.

John Harvey Kellogg, cornflake-pioneer, prophet of degeneracy theory and author of the 'thirty-nine signs' shown by masturbators. His list was so comprehensive as to damn the entire populace at a stroke. (CORBIS-BETTMANN/UPI)

Condoms from the mid-nineteenth century, printed with erotic scenes. (TOPHAM)

An advertisement for birth-control devices printed in Dr H. A. Allbutt's *The Wife's Handbook*, first published in 1886. It would be nearly another hundred years before contraception truly liberated women. (TOPHAM)

Section Three: The Sexual Self

Cartoon by R. Chast for the *New Yorker* magazine, printed shortly after the discovery of the 'gay gene' had been announced. (ROZ CHAST/NEW YORKER COLLECTION)

Drag queens at a Gay Pride rally. Could gender identity really be inscribed in the brain? (TRIP/S. GRANT)

A breastfeeding mother. The way she relates to her baby may profoundly influence its own attachment styles later in life. (TELEGRAPH COLOUR LIBRARY)

Gender play: boys tend to gravitate towards 'masculine' and aggressive toys like trucks and guns. (SANDY FELSENTHAL/CORBIS)

Girls, meanwhile, prefer dolls and more 'inclusive' activities. But how much of this behaviour is inborn and how much learned as children grow up? (JENNIE WOODCOCK/CORBIS)

Bestiality has been a part of sexual experimentation in many cultures. It is graphically illustrated in carvings on the Lakshmana temple in Khajuraho, India. (TRIP/H. ROGERS)

Elaborations on the basic theme: small ads from a men's porn magazine.

Whitney Houston – the most beautiful woman in the world? (BILL DAVILA/RETNA)

The young Marlon Brando – the most handsome man? (CORBIS-BETTMANN/UPI)

'36–24–36': study of waist-to-hip ratio in women by Devendra Singh. Singh found a direct correlation between low waist-to-hip ratios, attractiveness and the ability to bear children – all over the world. (DEVENDRA SINGH/APA)

Waist-to-hip ratio taken to its extreme: a severe corset from the mid-nineteenth century. (HULTON DEUTSCH/CORBIS)

Men inhale female copulines in an experiment by Astrid Jütte. It demonstrates the importance of odour as one of the most sophisticated and subtle of our sexual signalling systems. (OPTOMEN TV)

Mangaia, southernmost of the Cook Islands. Was this a place devoted to pleasure yet devoid of romantic attachment? Or merely an illustration of the West's obsession with love? (DENNIS MARSICO/CORBIS)

Plato, one of the most influential of the ancient Greek philosophers, who pictured love as an incredibly finely-tuned mechanism which inspired us to seek, recognise and respond to the very person with whom we truly deserved to be joined. (GIANNI DAGLI ORTI/CORBIS)

Tristan and Isolde: one of the great romantic myths of the Western world. (MARY EVANS PICTURE LIBRARY)

The Capilano suspension bridge near Vancouver: scene of an unusual experiment by Donald Dutton and Art Aron, who tried to prove the importance of anxiety in sexual attraction. (TRIP/R. STYLES)

Intriguing evidence for the Narcissus effect. When shown various faces, people sometimes choose a sex-changed version of their own as the most attractive. (PERCEPTION LABORATORY/UNIVERSITY OF ST ANDREWS)

Marriage counselling, the modern way. Psychologist John Gottman observes as a couple discuss an area of continuing conflict in their marriage while wired up to an array of technological equipment. (OPTOMEN TV)

Preface

'Boys are made to squirt and girls are made to lay eggs. And if the truth be known, boys don't very much care what they squirt into.' Gore Vidal looked up over the rim of his coffee cup and smiled. 'Put that in your book, why don't you?'

We were taking a break during the filming of a television series about the American presidency and Vidal was being his usual mischievous self. At the time, I was a good way into the first draft of this book, and while half of me agreed with him, the other half could not have disagreed more. Most men care enormously what they squirt into, even at their most aroused, and women don't lay eggs for just anyone. Moreover, alongside the evolutionary drive to reproduce to which Vidal was presumably alluding, there are also enormous cultural influences on sexuality, and these have often shaped us just as decisively. Until 1861, for example, homosexual behaviour was a hanging offence in England, and in the United States it was considered a psychiatric disorder until only two decades ago, at which point, as the neuroscientist Simon LeVay wittily remarks, 'twenty million homosexuals gained immediate cure'. Many of these individuals desired only those of their own sex, yet the threat of execution or stigmatisation led many to believe they were damned or diseased, creating a sense of fear which affected them to the innermost parts of their being.

The full force of cultural pressures, however, has traditionally been foisted upon women. Designed by natural selection as the seed-bearers for the human race, they have been subject to almost maniacal supervision, their movements curtailed and their desires often cruelly suppressed. Indeed, I can think of only one place where women have enjoyed something approaching total sexual freedom: the little village of Nagyrev in Eastern Europe during the First World War. And as we'll see in Chapter 2, it's a strange exception indeed.

Human societies the world over are stuffed with morals, laws and religious beliefs which circumscribe and often radically redirect the sexuality of their citizens. Yet in the eight years during which I've been writing and making television programmes about sex, I've also come to recognise that there's far more to its overall constitution than either 'nature' or 'culture'. There's the all-important 'nurture' as well.

On one occasion, I found myself working with the family and ex-colleagues of Jeffrey Dahmer, the Milwaukee serial killer who dismembered and had sex with the body parts of young men. On another, I was interviewing a female necrophile, an auto-erotic asphyxiator and an elderly man interested only in above-the-knee amputees. Overridingly, these individuals led me to appreciate the impact on our sexuality of various physical and psychological factors, acting on us during our formative years in the womb and the world.

And so, considering all these forces together, it seemed to me that human sexuality was forged by three interlocking principles: our basic evolutionary drives, the laws and beliefs of our culture, and the particularities of our own individual make-up, both mental and physical. Nature, culture, and nurture.

This book is an attempt to consider these three principles in unison, to strip sexuality down to its component parts and examine how they function and fit together. It would be impossible to explore some of the most complex issues in the fullness they deserve, so I have tried to make the text as clear as possible while providing a reasonably full bibliography for those who wish to pursue any topics further. My main hope is to have assembled and considered, as accurately as I can, what I perceive to be the major threads in a topic which is of vital interest to everyone and which is still too little understood.

Many people have helped in this undertaking. My most frequent correspondence has been with the academics and writers whose theories and findings have made up the bulk of the research; so numerous that I have thanked them in a separate section. A big thank-you also goes to Peter Gillbe, on whose wisdom, patience and friendship I have relied (as always) heavily; to Sara Ramsden, whose clear head and constant enthusiasm have been a joy; to Richard Curson Smith, a good friend and great debating partner; to Kate Roach and Charlotte Butler (thanks, Kate, for saving me from some embarrassing errors); and in particular to Polly Hope, who has collaborated on many sections of the manuscript and whose tireless, expert work is shown throughout. You've been brilliant, Polly, as I hope you know.

I'd also like to thank my agent, Jonny Geller, for his faith and continual encouragement; Araminta Whitley, who helped me believe I could write this book in the first place; Alan Samson at Little, Brown, who was brave enough to take it on, and Andrew Gordon, for his patient and painstaking editing. Thanks also to Linda Silverman for her picture research and to Matthew Rock, who provided early and much-needed support. Throughout the process of trying to put words on paper — easily the most frustrating part — I've been helped many times by my family; in particular by my mother, Virginia Andreae, by my brothers Giles, Hugo and Tobyn, and by my parents-in-law, Michael and Sandra Beer. To my late father, John Andreae, who saw the book commissioned but not completed, I also owe so much.

Finally, my most heartfelt thanks go to my wife Lisa, who was busy incubating our first son Jacob for most of the time I was writing, and who has recently given birth to our second, Jonah. She gave me the courage to get started, the will to carry on, and more love, support and sound advice (editorial and otherwise) than a grouchy, often distracted husband could possibly have hoped for, let alone deserved.

I am a man, I count nothing human foreign to me.

Terence (*c.* 190–159 BC)

PART ONE

BASIC INSTINCTS

*The fundamental characteristics of male and female
sexual desire. How they evolved and why they differ.*

1

Men

Three thousand miles off the north-east coast of New Zealand, adrift in the middle of the Pacific, lies the tiny island of Pitcairn. Two miles long and just over a mile wide, Pitcairn is still a British colony, and its fifty inhabitants are the legacy of a startling natural experiment which strikes at the heart of the male sexual condition.

Just over two hundred years ago, in 1790, fifteen men and thirteen women landed on this otherwise uninhabited island and set about creating a new life. Nine of the men were mutineers from Captain Bligh's ill-fated *Bounty* voyage; the rest were Polynesian women and their partners.

The party was led by Fletcher Christian, once Bligh's trusted mate, who, for the nine months since the mutiny, had been scouring the seas for a suitable place to bring his hijacked vessel and her increasingly fretful crew to rest. Navigating the *Bounty* into Pitcairn's waters, Christian at last thought he had found a safe haven. The land seemed rich and fertile, the climate was temperate, and the craggy rocks which formed the shoreline were guaranteed to dissuade all but the most determined of visitors. What's more, the only existing records of Pitcairn put it two hundred miles further east.

Jubilant at their discovery, the mutineers scrambled ashore and scaled the rocks to a green area where the land began to level out. Two hundred feet up, surrounded by wild fruits and trees, with their women beside them and the uncharted sea all around, Christian and his colleagues must have felt like the first men on Earth. Here, in their new Eden, they would set about building a new life unencumbered by government or religion. Each mutineer would have a house, a woman, and a plot of land. Other than that, there would be no laws, and no artificial constraints on pleasure.

Everyone was to do what came naturally, and they did. The men argued, fought and killed each other and the women were divided among the ever-dwindling number of victors.

First, the *Bounty*'s blacksmith, Jack Williams, stole a woman from her Polynesian lover Tararo in an effort to replace his own wife, who had fallen from a cliff while collecting birds' eggs. In response, the six Polynesian men made two retaliatory raids. The first was unsuccessful, resulting in the deaths of two of their own number. The second was more productive, providing them with the scalps of four mutineers and the potential to capture their four wives. But then the Polynesians fell to arguing over who should take charge of one of the women, Teraura. Teimua, who believed it should be him, began wooing her with songs. But Minarii, who disagreed, picked up a musket and blew out Teimua's brains.

Of the two remaining Polynesian men, one had his head split with an axe when he tried to climb into bed with the widow of the murdered Brown, and the other was hunted down and shot by a rage-fuelled Edward Young. The four remaining mutineers divided the women more or less equally between them, until the irksome Quintal lost his drinking companion McKoy (who had thrown himself from a cliff) and decided to stir up trouble by stealing Young's second consort, Mauatua. Young (who was in league with the other remaining mutineer, Adams) decided to act first and invited Quintal over for a drink, plied him with liquor until he could barely stand, then felled him with an axe.

Of the fifteen men who had landed on the island, only two would live to see the new century. And in 1800, Young also died, from asthma. In the ten years they had been there, twelve men had been murdered, one had committed suicide, and one was being buried by the last remaining survivor, John Adams. The last sailor, still aged only thirty-six, looked around with supreme disconsolation at the chaos which had been wrought by both his party and the Polynesians, his only comfort the ten women who had made it unscathed through the bloodshed and the twenty children who had come into his care.

Demise of the noble savage

The tale of Pitcairn is just one of many stories about what happens when people are taken out of the natural context of their lives and placed on a desert island to fend for themselves. From *Robinson Crusoe* to *Lord of the Flies*, such stories have held particular allure because they grapple with some of the most fundamental questions underpinning our lives. When stripped of all comforts, without the sanctions of religion, the guiding hand of the law or the well-trodden path of custom, what would we really be like? What if there were no one to punish us when we were bad, and no one to praise or advance us when we were good? Would we hold our selfish impulses in check and act for the benefit of all? Or would we be tempted to violate our most dearly-held moral codes at the earliest opportunity?

Novelists, philosophers and – in more recent times – social scientists have debated this issue from as many angles and with as many theories as there are examples to illustrate them. But nowhere was the debate more heated than in the drawing rooms of eighteenth-century Europe, at just about the time the *Bounty* first set sail.

In one camp were the followers of the English philosopher Thomas Hobbes, who believed that man was essentially a selfish, warlike creature whose baser impulses must be held in check by civilisation and societal control. Without these, Hobbes had declared, the life of man would be 'solitary, brutish, and short', with everyone living 'in continual fear and danger of violent death'.

In contrast, the French thinker Jean-Jacques Rousseau was a staunch believer in man's natural goodness, and proposed that civilisation corrupted an otherwise 'noble savage'. If only we could rid ourselves of culture and return to a 'state of nature', Rousseau held that, free of 'civilising' laws, human vice and misery would disappear and we would be left innocent and happy.

It was a heavy blow to the followers of Rousseau when news of the ultimate fate of the *Bounty* mutineers reached British shores in the early nineteenth century, especially when the story of their collective demise was broadcast in language as colourful as that used by the Reverend Thomas Boyles Murray. His bestselling interpretation of the expedition, *Pitcairn: The Island, the People and the Pastor*, painted the mutineers as no better or worse than the average human, merely men who, 'removed from the restraints imposed upon the wicked . . . showed in their hearts the workings of the depraved heart of man'.

Feuding, jealousy, and murder. Bitter power-struggles with continual outbreaks of violence. The subjugation and exploitation of whichever party was vulnerable. And at the root of it all, male sexual competition over women, with permanent access to the greatest number as each man's ultimate goal. More pressing than peace, more urgent than prosperity, more powerful than life itself. The picture which emerged here was the opposite of what Rousseau would have painted and as bleak as anything envisioned by Hobbes. It was nasty, but was it true?

The first spark of life

To appreciate the source of human sexual motivation, whether Man's or Woman's, we need to travel back beyond the origins of our early ancestors, beyond the origins of male and female, beyond even the origins of sex, to the origins of life itself. It was only six years after the first publication of Murray's book that one man would attempt to do just that, and in terms which would ignite controversy the world over.

Charles Darwin had failed at two careers, one as a doctor and the other as a clergyman, before he became a naturalist, set sail aboard the *Beagle*, circumnavigated the globe, and began to plot his first revolutionary masterpiece, *On the Origin of Species by Means of Natural Selection*. Having noticed on his voyage the underlying similarities between many different types of species, both living and extinct, Darwin began to speculate that all animals might originally have come from some common source, multiplying and diverging through the slow march of time to suit their different environments.

At a time when received wisdom had it that the world had been created in 4004 BC, by a man with a white beard who had given life to all creatures at the same time and then made man to supervise them, Darwin's view was labelled a heresy. 'Let us hope it is not true,' whispered the wife of the Bishop of Worcester, 'but if it is, let us pray it does not become generally known.' Unfortunately for her, and for all who believed in a six-day creation spree, a rib, and a ripe apple, it was and it did; only today we know a little more about the circumstances and a lot more about the process. And when we accept its implications, the Pitcairn story will seem a lot more credible.

The distinguished British biologist John Maynard Smith sits crouched in his deep, worn armchair. Postcards with dirty jokes about peacocks (a collector's item among biologists) adorn the walls of his dusty green-grey office, while foreign covers of his major works are sellotaped to the back of the door. Maynard Smith is one of three contemporary biologists who, between them, have elaborated and expanded Darwin's insights into a comprehensive and sophisticated theory which accounts for the origin, development and nature of all living organisms, from the first and simplest bacteria to the most complex multi-celled creatures, including humans.

Maynard Smith's co-conspirators are George Williams, whose stooping figure and furrowed brow give him more than a passing resemblance to Abraham Lincoln; and Robert Trivers, an eccentric genius from Rutgers University, New York. They are not without their disagreements, nor are they the only scientists to have contributed to the debate, but their story is strong and compelling and provides the best account we have so far of why we exist, how we got here, and what we're really like.

Three and a half billion years ago, the Earth was a lifeless, turbulent cauldron racked by lightning and swept by racing winds. There were no trees on this Earth; no plants or grass or fields. By today's standards, this planet was positively hostile, a hellish soup of sulphur and acids, but around and within its surface were all the elements needed to generate the first forms of life: carbon, phosphorus, and hydrogen. The only thing required was the right kind of kick-start.

Then, bolts of ancient lightning struck the Earth's surface, carbon, hydrogen and oxygen were fused together, and eventually the first amino acids were formed. In the sequence of events that would lead to life, these amino acids were crucial since, clustering around sugar phosphate backbones to improve their stability, they developed the power to reproduce. The first such acid was RNA (ribonucleic acid), with DNA (deoxyribonucleic acid) following some time later. Over the next billion years, unimaginably large numbers of different combinations of DNA and RNA came together, some of which were better at reproducing themselves than others. Through the incremental process of trial and error, those that were successful endured into subsequent generations, while those that were not were wiped out.

At the end of this period, one of the most successful combinations turned out to be several long strands of DNA which had grouped together and hidden within a protective membrane of fats. This was the origin of the cell, and bacteria, the first single-celled creatures, emerged.

Once again, some bacteria were better equipped to reproduce than others, with whatever contributed to successful reproduction being passed down the line to subsequent generations. Then, some two billion years ago, something radical happened to the reproductive process which would have far-reaching effects and allow for the development of a greater and more sophisticated range of organisms than had ever been possible before. That something was sex.

Instead of taking on the task of reproduction alone, producing exact copies of themselves again and again, some forms of life began to work together, in pairs. Each would donate a copy of their genetic material and the brew would be mixed together to produce a third organism – the offspring – which, though similar to each of its parents, was also different from both. These 'hybrids' were the first and simplest sexually reproduced creatures on Earth, no larger nor more complex than a cell. Yet despite their apparent simplicity, something amazing had taken place. Sex, the simple act of mixing DNA, had been born. And from that moment on, there was no looking back.

'Imagine a tree which produces both sexual and asexual seeds.' George Williams, who has a singular gift for metaphor, uses this analogy to explain how, once created, sex would endure to become the most robust and successful form of reproduction on Earth. Williams believes that in an entirely predictable environment, where everything ran like clockwork and nothing ever changed, sex would actually be at a disadvantage when compared with earlier forms of reproduction, like cloning. Cloning is much more efficient. It only takes one parent, all the offspring are the same, and the energy saved by not having to seek a partner can be spent on producing more children. Indeed, asexual species typically breed at far higher rates than sexual ones. However, in conditions where the climate varies, where predators are constantly learning new tricks, and where nothing can be taken for granted, sex is a godsend. For the continually varying organisms it creates makes it likely that some, at least, will be impregnable to whatever predators, parasites, storms or famines a hostile Earth might throw at them.

And the early Earth, for all its bounty, was not without hazards. As the number of organisms on the planet grew, some found food sources conducive to their survival within others, leading to a continual war between parasite and prey. Large creatures preyed on small ones and small ones on microbial ones, with the microbes fighting back by parasitising their predators from the inside. It wasn't so much a food chain as a free-for-all. Nor were other organisms the only threat. The Earth, which had brought forth life, had the power to destroy it, too. Earthquakes, meteors, floods, tempests, the bitter winter winds and several ice ages have all played their part in extinguishing as many life-forms as those that have been nurtured and sustained.

Thus, in the case of Williams' tree, where both varied sexual and identical asexual seeds are fighting for space, for cover, and for food, it is the sexual ones who will win out. They may not be as numerous or as uniform as their asexual brethren, and many of them may be weaker, but some at least will happen to possess genetic combinations that render them immune to winter, invisible to hungry birds, or improbably skilled at sucking water from the ground.

Sex, therefore, gradually began to overtake cloning as the preferred form of reproduction among most species. With the endless array of unique combinations it created, new possibilities appeared all the time. And eventually, as the most successful proliferated and diversified, they developed more and more sophisticated ways to promote their own survival, gathering into complex multi-celled structures with protective armour, subtle camouflage, and highly advanced food-gathering devices. Some, looking for ever more crafty ways to survive, even decided to make the next great leap into the swirling waters of evolution. Not just sex, but gender.

John Maynard Smith believes the answer to the question of gender lies in specialisation. If two members of the same species were to develop different forms, they would be better at different reproductive tasks. In fact, this specialisation is what being male or female is all about, with the male baldly defined as the organism which produces small, mobile sex cells (sperm) which swim to the egg, and the female the organism which produces large, nutrient-filled ones (eggs) which can sustain the new foetus. But although this explains why we have inherited two sexes rather than one or one hundred, it doesn't explain why one should contribute so much more than the other.

The big question about gender, from a biological point of view, is: why males? At first they don't appear to make much sense. Without being too judgemental about it, they seem to contribute little more to the act of reproduction than their own DNA. No food for the foetus, no womb in which it can develop, and none of the burdensome process of pregnancy, nesting or weaning which females of most species are obliged to undertake. Why did any female allow it? Why didn't she hold back until she found a similarly equipped partner who was prepared to share the burden equally?

The reason lies in a substance contained within the tail of the sperm and the cytoplasm of the egg, known as organelles. These are what propel the sperm towards the egg, but although they make a great engine, they are not strictly necessary for the act of reproduction. Moreover, if the egg allowed them in, they would almost certainly be tempted to fight with the egg's own organelles, weakening or destroying the offspring. As a result, sperm and egg came to a compromise, with the former agreeing to leave everything except the DNA needed for reproduction outside the ovum wall. No organelles, no tail. In this respect, the male's lack of contribution was in fact his greatest asset. And as long as he could find a partner who was willing to provide enough food for both, everyone was happy. This, therefore, is why we have inherited not just any old combination of sexes, but the specific binary complement of male and female that characterises the members of almost all sexually reproducing species.

And with the most successful males and females mating and passing their mixed genes down to future generations, nature now had a continual proliferation of new and varied organisms from which to sculpt her choices. And the question of which would multiply and which would be eliminated depended, as ever, on their success at the task of reproduction. Organisms which were unsuited to the task withered and died; organisms which succeeded spread, diversified and multiplied, developing ever more sophisticated weapons to promote their own survival and enhance their reproductive efficiency.

Gradually, and with ever-increasing complexity, fish evolved, then amphibians, reptiles, birds, and finally mammals. But essentially, for all their elaboration, efficiency, and even beauty, all these different life-forms remained geared to one task and one task only: passing their genes down through the generations in the greatest numbers and with the greatest rate of success. This is the origin of skeletons and skin, of veins and arteries, of internal organs, muscles, limbs and brains. But evolution has not just shaped bodies. In humans, it is also the origin of thought and movement, of plan and fantasy, and of our dreams and desires. Whether we like it or not, we, like all living creatures, are basically machines for maximising our own reproductive success, living out a design which has evolved over the three and a half billion years since that flash of lightning gave rise to the first spark of life.

In the simplest terms, this means that our bodies and our brains must have been fashioned according to three interlocking principles of design:

first, to make us want sex with the best possible mates; second, to ensure our own survival so that we can do so; and third, to protect and provide for our offspring.

In a species made up of differently equipped sexes, different mating specialisations would naturally accrue. And this is where the last of our trio of biologists, Robert Trivers, comes in. Looking at the harsh facts of sexual reproduction, Trivers produced a landmark paper in 1972 which attempted to unravel the mysteries of mate choice by looking at the costs of parenthood. In all living beings, he suggested, the time and energy put into making sex cells, seeking and having sex, gestating the young and rearing them to maturity, could be most usefully seen as an investment by each parent in its own reproductive success. Breeding, he went on to speculate, is simply too exhausting to be taken lightly. Whichever sex is obliged to invest the most in its offspring, therefore, is very likely to be the sex which chooses its partners most carefully.

As we've already seen, male sex cells – sperm – are small, mobile and very easy to produce. Because they're so small and don't have to be packed with nutrients, they can be made in dizzying numbers. The average human male is capable of replacing his sperm at a rate of three million per minute, meaning that each man could technically produce enough sperm to inseminate every single woman on the planet – if they were to agree. So, by Trivers's logic, they can and should be spread around as widely as possible. All that's absolutely required from a male to produce a new human is a few minutes of sex culminating in ejaculation. Beyond that, any parental contribution is entirely voluntary. When set against the heavy and unavoidable costs for women – the manufacture of eggs, the nine months of draining pregnancy, and the further years of breast-feeding and care – the parental investment demanded from men is virtually nil. If fatherhood is so undemanding, what should stop men going all out to seek and have sex with as many partners as possible? After all, they lose very little and stand to gain a great deal.

Trivers's theory might sound like a just-so story, finding a dubious rationale for rampant male philandering in a rather too-neat evolutionary package. But the elegance and worth of his ideas are borne out more conclusively when we look at the very few species where males contribute a great deal to rearing the young. Among seahorses, and over thirty species of birds, while females produce the eggs, males do most of the rearing; and sure enough, it's the males who are choosier about their mates and the females who have to compete to catch their eye. And we'll see later on, wherever we look, that whenever it seems that males will have to invest more in their offspring, they become visibly more concerned with the quality of their sexual partners.

For the most part, however, Trivers's message for human sexual strategies is straightforward and ruthless. Contributing little more to the act of reproduction than small, highly mobile packages of DNA, men would profit most from being driven to compete fiercely for access to women, then by mating prodigiously with as many as possible. Seen in this light, perhaps the surprise of the Pitcairn story is not that it escalated into a spiralling series of wife-stealings and murders, but that these activities do not form a much greater part of the fabric of human relations. Unless, of course, they do.

Sex lives of the ancients

Laura Betzig, an ebullient Darwinian anthropologist at the University of Michigan, has spent the last ten years investigating the history of the male sex drive. The Pitcairn story doesn't surprise her at all. Wherever there have been resources to accumulate and land to dominate, Betzig holds that men have fought fiercely for supremacy, then directed their energies towards accumulating and enjoying the maximum number of women. In the early empires, where feudalism and slavery laid the groundwork for capture and confinement, the figures reached dizzying heights.

King Hammurabi of Babylon kept several hundred 'slave wives'; the Aztec and Inca kings more than four thousand; the Chinese emperor Fei-ti ten thousand; and emperor Udayama of India more than sixteen thousand, in quarters ringed with fire and guarded by palace eunuchs.

So much for the despotic ancient civilisations. Here, where ruthlessness had once been the surest guarantee of survival, the least a king's people could do was to ensure that their leader was adequately provisioned with the pleasures obtaining from power – women among them. Their continued well-being might depend on it. But what about the urbanity and much-vaunted refinement of the Roman and subsequent European empires? Here, surely, Betzig would find male sexuality characterised by greater equanimity and restraint. Her answer was a resounding 'no'.

A quick roll-call of the twelve Caesars of Rome finds Julius drawing up a bill to legitimise his union 'with any woman, or women, he pleased', while his successor, Augustus, 'harboured a passion for deflowering girls, who were collected for him from every quarter, even by his wife'. Tiberius' lusts were 'worthy of an Oriental tyrant'; Caligula 'surpassed his predecessor's licentiousness'; Claudius was 'extremely passionate'; while the sixth Caesar, Nero, was a picture of wantonness and debauchery who would tie women to the stake and 'satisfy his brutal lust under the appearance of devouring parts of their bodies'. Relatively little is written about the seventh, eighth and ninth Caesars, though Galba is described as brutal and greedy and Otho and Vitellius as 'the two most despicable men in the whole world by reason of their unclean, idle, and pleasure-loving lives'. The final three, making up the twelve, were Vespasian and his two sons Titus and Domitian. While Vespasian contented himself with an afternoon nap in the company of 'one of the several mistresses whom he had engaged', Titus and Domitian had less mainstream inclinations. According to the strait-laced and ever-reproachful historian of their peccadilloes, Suetonius, the former consorted with a 'troop of inverts and eunuchs' while the latter 'was profligate and lewd towards women and boys alike' and 'referred to his constant sexual activities as "bed wrestling", as though it was a sport'.

So there we have it. The twelve Caesars were not so much the glorious leaders of a sober and powerful state as a group of sexual gluttons who had clawed their way to the top, grabbed the talent, and enjoyed it to the full. Far from the grave solidity of their statues, they were a bunch of beasts in togas.

With the benefit of hindsight, the stability provided by democracy, and a long-standing policy of monogamy, it's easy to ridicule the primitive antics of these early hedonists; wide-eyed children treating their empires like toy-cupboards. We're wiser, smarter, more self-disciplined now. Two thousand years of Christian teaching and temperance have made us more restrained and moderate. Or have they?

After looking at Rome, Betzig turned her attention to medieval Christendom, where all was not as squeaky clean as it seemed. Inspired after the Crusades by tales of Oriental harems, medieval nobles constructed their castles with specially secluded women's quarters, known as *gynaecea*, whose residents were encouraged to while away the hours playing games and making shirts, waiting for a call from their master. Even those paragons of Christian morality, the popes, were not exempt. The image of papal chastity was beginning to crack as early as AD 440, when Pope Sixtus II was tried for seducing a nun, and from that moment on it was nearly all downhill. John XII, who was Pontiff between 955 and 964, was said to have had sex with his mother, his niece, his father's concubines and many noblemen's wives; John XXIII (1410-15) was charged with 'having hired and maintained a sacrilegious intercourse with three hundred nuns'; while Alexander VI (1492-1503), better known by his birth-name Rodrigo Borgia, was perhaps the most infamous of all. Even before ascending to the throne, Borgia had suffered a severe reprimand from the usually mild Pope Pius II for attending an orgy with all the noble ladies and none of the men of Siena while wearing his official regalia (the regalia, not the orgy, was the problem). Borgia appeared to take no notice. As Pope, he never travelled without a troop of dancing girls, took twenty-five prostitutes into his quarters most nights, and arranged the infamous 'Joust of Whores', in which naked women were obliged to race on all fours down paths illuminated by candles, while Borgia and his friends attempted to mount whichever took their fancy.

In analysing Betzig's data of the early empires, the Romans, the medieval Christians and even rulers from more recent times, one could be forgiven for assuming that, given unbridled power, men overridingly direct it to two interlocking ends: the protection of their estate and the acquisition of women. Wherever one looks, and whatever they claim, the pattern seems to hold true. From the Pacific atolls to the Amazon jungles, from the wastelands of Waco to the royal palaces of Brunei, and from Tiananmen Square to the Playboy Mansion, women are the currency, the incentive, and the reward of power. 'All the money in the world,' remarked the one-time richest man in the world, Aristotle Onassis, 'would mean nothing without women.' Women in the plural, of course.

The adapted mind

There is, however, a problem here. Thus far, we've only been talking about the sex lives of leaders. Granted, they are useful because they show what men are capable of when they are above or beyond the legal restrictions which apply to most of us. But might there not be something about the nature of leadership itself which alters men's minds? Might there be something different about leaders *per se* which makes them an exceptional group, unrepresentative of the male community at large?

Enter two of the major players in the newest angle on sexual investigation, evolutionary psychology. John Tooby and Leda Cosmides share a startling, light-filled house in the hills above Santa Barbara, with a panoramic view over its sparkling Pacific shoreline. Refugees from the more conventional Harvard University where, in the mid-1980s, evolutionary psychology was considered heresy, Tooby and Cosmides preach their message with religious zeal. They suggest that, as all human hearts, or hands, or ears share a similar design, whether they belong to labourers or leaders, so all human minds are created with a similar set of programmes. This set of programmes has evolved according to the same selection pressures that have shaped every other organ of every other human body: chiefly, the pressure to reproduce as effectively as possible. In the case of the human male, where the primary strategy for reproductive success would seem to be frequent mating with a large number of female partners, Tooby and Cosmides expected to find evidence of mental programmes, or 'adaptations' as they call them, which encouraged them to do just that, no matter what their race, status, colour or creed. And their colleagues have not been slow at collecting the evidence.

With his former student Bruce Ellis, Donald Symons, the self-styled Grand Old Man of the evolutionary approach and another resident of Santa Barbara, set about issuing questionnaires to over four hundred students, aimed at uncovering the nature and extent of their sexual fantasies. These, he imagined, might give a truer picture of the strategies underpinning sexuality than did their actual behaviour. While in the real world sexual behaviour has to strike a compromise with the wishes of the opposite sex, the available resources, and the snarling male competition, in the world of fantasy all men have the power to do exactly as they please.

Symons found, in the case of men, that 30 per cent had fantasised about having sex with more than a thousand women, while more than half regularly switched partners during the course of a single fantasy. Asked to outline these, a typical male responded that he imagined being the mayor of a small town filled with nude girls between the ages of twenty and twenty-four. 'I like to take walks,' he reported, 'and pick out the best-looking one that day, and she engages in intercourse with me. All the women have sex with me any time I want.'

But sex takes time. If men, circumstances permitting, were able to enact such fantasies, they would need to have evolved specific adaptations which encouraged them to get on with the job as quickly as possible. How else could they get through such numbers? It was just such an adaptation that evolutionary psychologist David Buss set out to test in one of the group studies for which he has become renowned. Buss, a giant of a man with steely blue eyes and a bone-crushing handshake, asked all his college students what would be the minimum amount of time they would be prepared to spend with someone before going to bed with them. Most of the men found that a week or so was perfectly respectable, but almost half were just as happy with only an hour. Seen from this perspective, the old slogan 'So many girls, so little time' wasn't just an idle, arrogant joke. It summed up the male sexual dilemma.

A second way for evolution to encourage men to get through many women would be to make them eager to receive the attentions of more than one partner at a time. To examine this possibility, Glenn Wilson, a native of New Zealand who now works at the London Institute of Psychiatry, collaborated with one of Britain's most successful tabloid newspapers, the *Mirror*, in sampling the sexual fantasies of 788 British people of different ages and socio-economic groups. His results suggested that nearly 50 per cent of the men had fantasised at one time or another about group-sex scenarios. It's a statistic borne out by nearly all swingers' groups, who testify that it is almost always men rather than their wives who make the first contact and who are initially the most eager to participate.

Although the work done by Symons, Buss and Wilson is telling, certain studies have gone further and attempted to catch these male sexual adaptations with their pants down, so to speak. Two researchers have been particularly active in this area: Russell Clark and Brian Gladue.

Clark's experiment was extremely straightforward. He simply wished to test in practice the findings that researchers like Buss had found in theory: namely, that men possess an adaptation for minimising the time they wish to spend with a woman before going to bed with her. To this end, he and his colleague Elaine Hatfield assembled a group of attractive female research students and positioned them at discreet intervals on his college campus in Florida. The students were to approach male passers-by and start a conversation by saying, 'Hi, I've been noticing you around town lately and I find you very attractive.' Then, they were to ask them one of three questions: 'Would you go out tonight?', 'Will you come over to my apartment?' or 'Would you go to bed with me tonight?' In response, about 50 per cent of the men agreed to go on a date; 69 per cent agreed to go back to their questioner's room; while fully 75 per cent agreed to head straight for bed. More men were willing to have sex with a total stranger than to spend a social evening with her.

All the findings pointed to powerful mechanisms which motivate men to grasp every possible sexual opportunity. Aside from minimising the time spent with women, and being interested in opportunities for sex with several different partners at once, a third way to maximise a man's chances would be to make him find women increasingly attractive as opportunities for sex with them begin to slip away. Brian Gladue decided to test whether this might be the case by asking men to rate the attractiveness of female patrons at a bar in the American Midwest at three allotted times over the course of an evening: nine o'clock, ten-thirty, and midnight. It was, in effect, an attempt to prove scientifically the oft-quoted adage that the girls look prettier at closing time. Controlling for the effects of alcohol and making sure that his guinea pigs stayed in the bar for the duration of the experiment, Gladue had prepared the ground carefully, and his hunch paid off. Over the four hours they had been there, the men's average ratings increased by about 17 per cent, meaning that a woman who had been given a score of six out of ten at the beginning of the evening was likely to have been given a score of seven by the end.

So far, Tooby and Cosmides' idea that men may have evolved specific adaptations to make the most of their reproductive potential seems to be holding true. They fantasise about large numbers, they like the idea of sex with several partners at the same time, they attempt to minimise the time spent with each, and their desire increases in proportion as opportunities for sex slip away. What's more, these findings seem to hold up in the marketplace and around the world just as securely as in the laboratory or on the campus. Male-oriented pornography, with its endless supply of anonymous, pouting models, is specifically designed to appeal to a mentality which takes pleasure in variety. Editors testify that while their readers have their favourites, the sure-fire selling point is 'new talent'. And this isn't just an effect of rampant Western consumerism: in other parts of the globe, anthropologists continue to catalogue the upfront disclosures of men who are not bound by the cultural ideal of monogamy. When asked why he insisted on sleeping with such a wide range of partners rather than content himself with a single wife, one Muria tribesman from central India replied matter-of-factly, 'Who wants to eat the same vegetable every day?'

The problem of number

A different vegetable every day. Mayor of a town filled with nude girls. Harems stocked with endless supplies of women. The monotony of the male sexual ideal is matched only by its difficulty to achieve. Let's put aside for the moment two of the most significant barriers: the desires of women and the laws of the land. What's left is the sheer problem of number.

The human race has a sex ratio of approximately one to one. On the face of it, there should be a woman for every man, and vice versa. But when we remember that the male sexual template has been fine-tuned over more than a billion years to calibrate itself for maximum reproductive success, we shouldn't be surprised to find it preferentially attuned to women who might be fertile. As we'll discover in Chapter 5, both sexes have evolved an extraordinary variety of mechanisms designed to help them gauge the fertility of potential partners. But for the moment, let's state the obvious and surmise that women who are pregnant or past childbearing age are generally (although by no means universally) considered less sexually appealing than those who are not.

Add into the equation that women are fertile for fewer years than men, and the ratio of partners who are either available or desirable drops dramatically. Furthermore, if certain men have acquired the wherewithal to keep large numbers of women to themselves, as in the case of the early despots, it drops even more. As a result, if men were to have the slightest chance of achieving their sexual nirvana of endless willing women, they were going to be driven to compete. And competition is the second great driving force behind the basic sexual instincts of men.

On Pitcairn, sexual competition was raw and brutal, possibly augmented by the fact that the number of men and women who arrived on the island was unequal. Fifteen men to thirteen women. All it took was the death of one more female to tip an initially uneasy situation over into violence. Among the early despots, competition was just as fierce. But, as new research shows, competition occurs in almost all circumstances where males meet, often in less ferocious bouts and with less deadly results, yet competition nonetheless. It might seem to be about status, or money, or power. But how much of the perennial competition between men is rooted in the struggle for sexual success?

Brian Gladue noticed an interesting difference between the attitudes of men and women towards competition when he took them to his Cincinnati laboratory and explained an experiment he planned to undertake. Participants were to be selected in pairs and sat in separate rooms. Both were to watch for a light to come on. When they saw it, they were to press a button on the desk in front of them as fast as possible. The participant who pressed first was designated the winner and was allowed to administer an electric shock to the opponent in the other room.

To all the men, this seemed like an appealing idea. They lined up and participated eagerly, racing to press the buttons and administering shocks with glee. Most women, on the other hand, couldn't see the point. A large proportion refused to participate, and those who did seemed in no special hurry to press their buttons. Even when they did, they were generally unenthusiastic about electrifying their opponents. On the surface, none of this had anything to do with sexuality, until Gladue began to analyse the male competitors' hormone levels. Upon doing so, he discovered that those who competed most aggressively and administered the most powerful electric shocks were those who had the highest levels of the male sex hormone, testosterone. What's more, those levels rose even more when the competitors were informed of their victories.

That testosterone is the hormone primarily responsible for the male sex drive, no one seems to doubt. A crystalline solution produced by the Leydig cells of the testes, it flows around the body in regular pulsatile rhythms, peaking every fifteen minutes or so during a man's major reproductive years. Commonly believed to prime men to be ready for regular sex, testosterone has been used with some effect to treat those with abnormally low levels of desire. In tests carried out during the early 1990s, men with naturally low levels of testosterone were treated for six months with testosterone replacements, during which they reported significant increases in the duration of their erections, the frequency of their ejaculations, and the overall degree of their libido.

What has been less commonly recognised is the degree to which testosterone seems to be implicated in competition too. Nevertheless, in support of Gladue's finding that the most competitive men have the highest testosterone levels, psychologist James Dabb Jr has found that actors, entertainers, football players and high-court judges all appear to have higher levels than church ministers. And his discovery that testosterone levels seem to spurt in winners too now also finds support from other tests. In one study, researchers discovered that the testosterone levels of military cadets decreases during the early and depressing period of officer training, then increases dramatically at graduation. In another, testosterone levels in tennis players were found to increase in response to victory and dip at the signs of defeat.

What then of the relationship between them? Is the hormonal circuitry which governs this form of aggressive competitiveness distinct from the one which drives sexual desire, or are they somehow linked? Let's consider two strands of evidence: one from the world of transsexuality and one from the American college system.

Milo, Johnnie and Matt are San Francisco bikers. With their beefy biceps, sawn-off T-shirts and tattoos they look for all the world like biker boys. In a sense they are, but they're also F-to-Ms: genetic females who wish to adopt a male appearance and identity, and in order to do so they inject themselves with testosterone. It has several startling effects. The most noticeable to the outside observer are physical. The F-to-Ms develop well-defined muscles; hair starts growing on their faces; their voices deepen; their skin becomes coarse, and their clitorises start to grow, often to the size of small penises. But just as dramatic are the psychological effects.

Very soon after they receive the shots, F-to-Ms start to feel sexually aroused. But it's not the sort of arousal they used to feel when their endocrine system was chiefly under the influence of the female hormones oestrogen and progesterone. It's active, intense, and very pressing indeed. Visual stimuli, in particular, become more or less impossible to ignore, and the urge to act on feelings of arousal becomes more pronounced. They feel, in the words of Milo, 'kicked off the benches and on to the playing field, where you feel like running for touchdown'. F-to-Ms are careful to point out that their sex drive hasn't appeared from nowhere; they felt arousal and desire before the injections. What's changed is the *nature* of that desire. Where, previously, feelings of competitiveness and arousal were subtle and separate, now they're urgent, aggressive, and fused.

Todd Crosset, a sports management professor at the University of Massachusetts, found the playing-field metaphor even more apposite when he examined 107 cases of rape, attempted rape and unwanted groping at 30 schools in the National Collegiate Athletic Association. Figures from 1990 to 1993 showed that those heavily involved in athletics made up only 3 per cent of the general school population but carried out 19 per cent of the sexual assaults.

Both these examples suggest that male sexuality and aggressive male competition may be linked, and from an evolutionary point of view, this seems to make some sense. If, through most of our past, the clearest route to reproductive success was to mate with many women, and if there was an imbalance between the number of women available for sex and the number of men trying to have sex with them, why not fit males with a single all-purpose gasoline that encouraged them to fight as hard as possible for access to those women, then, if they won, to be ready and primed to mate?

More controversially, some investigators have suggested that testosterone's dual purpose has blurred competition and desire together at all stages of the male sexual strategy. Testosterone-fuelled aggression might be directed not just at males but at unwilling females too. What would be the point in overcoming the competition if the prize herself refused to yield? Seen in this light, could Todd Crosset's sportsmen rapists simply be high-testosterone, dominant males living out *in extremis* a sexual programme which lurks within all males?

The suggestion that there may be something of the rape mentality underlying all male sexuality is explosive. For the last three decades, feminist writers such as Susan Brownmiller have been developing arguments that rape is about domination and power rather than sex. It is perpetrated, the argument runs, by a patriarchal society wishing to continue the subjugation of women through a reign of hostility and terror. But the more the motivation behind rape is examined, the more it appears to contain a certain kind of brutal evolutionary logic. If the final aim of male sexuality is to reproduce as widely as possible, female consent is, on one level at least, irrelevant.

Neil Malamuth, of the University of California in Los Angeles, has studied the causes of rape for more than two decades and concedes that, when combined with other personality factors, it is the evolved sexual mechanisms in the minds of men which set the stage for the occurrence of what he calls 'coercive sexuality'. He suggests that because of their greater capacity for impersonal sex, men can be fully sexually functional in the face of an unwilling sexual partner. However, Malamuth is careful to point out the limitations of an evolutionary approach. The simple fact remains that in the real world, all men are not rapists – whether or not they might wish to be. Rape, he emphasises, is not an inevitable consequence of evolution; it has plenty to do with power as well.

Numerous studies have with conflicting results tried to elicit whether the rape mentality truly does underlie most male sexual desire. Those who argue that it does point to the high proportion of men reporting rape fantasies, to the considerable success of pornographic material depicting rape scenarios (there is a series of comics and videos in Japan devoted to the exploits of a character called Rapeman), and to the epidemics of rape in wartime, when legal sanctions cannot be applied. Those who disagree point out that many gang and wartime rapes are perpetrated with bottles or rifles rather than penises, that oral and anal rape is frequent, and the victims are as frequently elderly or male as they are young or potentially fertile. In many cases the victims may also be killed after the rape. Surely this cannot be the product of sexual mechanisms which ought to hone in on potential chances to reproduce?

In reality, the causes of rape are more complex than either of these positions suggest, requiring a multi-dimensional understanding which also takes into account the family dynamic in which the offender has been raised; the particular constellation of genetic attributes with which he has been born; his society's attitude towards women and towards rape; and a number of neurological and psychiatric possibilities too. But even if the theorists who hold that rape grows out of basic male adaptations have grasped one aspect of the truth, then why are more men not rapists? To answer that question, we need to know a little more about the structure of the human brain.

Intellectual faculties and animal propensities

In the 1940s and 1950s, the celebrated neuroscientist Paul MacLean advanced a theory of the brain which pictured it as a three-part hierarchy. Right at the core was the primitive reptilian tier, centring around the brain stem. This dealt with the simplest bodily reflexes: breathing, heart-rate regulation, and movement. Surrounding this reptilian brain was the paleo-mammalian brain, also called the limbic system, which was inherited from our earliest mammal ancestors and dealt with deep and strong emotional reactions, which would have aided our survival: fear, anger, elation and sexual desire. And finally, forming an outer casing over almost the whole surface of the brain, was the neo-mammalian brain, also known as the cortex – the grey matter which allows us to think, remember, understand and communicate. These three interlocking systems, inherited from different stages in our evolution, combined into one composite whole, which MacLean christened the 'triune brain'.

While all mammals shared a similarly designed limbic system, MacLean noted, only higher mammals had developed the larger outgrowth of grey matter that surrounds it, the all-important frontal cortex. And it was the cortex, he reasoned, with its capacity for language, logic, and long-term planning, which held the basic instinctual desires of the limbic system in check. Raw evidence of the true limbic drives lurking underneath the cortex was not easy to find, and would come from some unlikely sources.

The underbelly of sexual history reveals a pattern of association between aggression and sex, those lurking drives of the limbic system, which is as constant as it is puzzling. Anthropologist Helen Fisher finds a primal link between them whenever she asks people about their most secret sexual desires. 'Ask women what they really fantasise about,' she slyly suggests, 'and two patterns keep repeating: romance and being bitten.' Fisher is being deliberately provocative, but the anthropological record reveals a grain of truth in her remark. The classic Indian sex manual of the third century AD, the *Kama Sutra*, recommends biting as a fine way to arouse one's partner, describing in detail five particular styles, while nineteenth- and early-twentieth-century anthropologists studying the so-called 'primitive cultures' sent back reports in which aggression in sex seemed to be the norm rather than the exception. 'Poking a finger in the eye counts as affection,' wrote one, describing the South American Sirionó people, 'and couples emerged with scars after passionate encounters.'

Another strand of evidence was unearthed around a hundred years before MacLean advanced his theory, with the unwitting aid of a railway worker named Phineas P. Gage. Gage was the foreman of a gang of railway workers near the town of Cavendish, in Vermont, during the 1850s. A popular and responsible leader, he was levelling the ground for a new piece of track when an unplanned explosion blew a three-foot iron bar clean through his skull. Gage was thrown on to his back, his body convulsing and jerking, and was swiftly carried to his hotel, where he was attended by a Dr John Harlow. Amazingly, Gage was sufficiently aware to explain what had happened, even pointing to the hole and saying, 'The iron bar entered here and passed through my head.' He then became feverish and lost consciousness.

In the days immediately following the incident, the prognosis did not look good. Fungus started growing from the hole in Gage's head; his friends implored Harlow to let him die. But the doctor continued to bathe his fevered patient, anxious to save his life and fascinated, despite himself, to see what would happen if he did. For the iron bar had torn right through the front of Gage's head, while leaving the deeper parts completely intact.

Slowly, Gage began to recover, and after a month of non-stop nursing, Harlow released him, anxious to see the result. He did not have to wait long. Gage was dismissed from his job because 'the equilibrium . . . between his intellectual faculties and animal propensities, seems to have been destroyed'. He became wilful, obstinate and unrealistic, dreaming up escapades and adventures that were no sooner devised than abandoned. He turned to drinking and brawling. He ran away from his wife, embarked upon a string of unsuccessful affairs, fell in and out of brothels, and finally died in 1861 after a series of epileptic convulsions.

At first, Gage's story had seemed like a miracle, but it turned out to be a tragedy. Without the controlling influences of the frontal cortex, his instinctual impulses had been unleashed – and they combined brute sexual desire with urgent, often hostile impetuosity.

Peter Fenwick finds the Gage story fascinating. A Professor of Psychiatry based at the Maudsley Hospital in London, Fenwick is a tall, stooping, kindly figure with a purposeful gait and large, steady hands. He is also one of the country's leading experts on epilepsy. Although Fenwick has never come across a case like Gage's, he has noticed a strong correlation between certain forms of epilepsy and highly increased levels of sexual desire. In the case of epileptic seizures of the frontal lobes in particular, Fenwick has had many patients ringing him up in despair, as their normal home lives are ruined by two- to three-day bursts of intense sexual feelings and the urge to go out and act on them. Then, as the convulsions subside, so their sexuality returns to normal, and their lives are continued, more or less peaceably, until the next time.

Fenwick believes that just as Gage's frontal cortex was damaged, so the cortices of his epileptic patients are temporarily knocked out of action, causing the limbic desires to rise to the surface and seek expression. But Fenwick feels that sexuality and aggression are not inextricably joined. Rather, they exist in very close proximity, with sexuality focused in the hypothalamus, and aggression seething away below it in a small area known as the amygdala. In this scheme of things, male sexuality and aggression co-exist in discrete but neighbouring positions within the human limbic system. They're fuelled by the same major hormone and capable of confusion, but are kept in check by the much larger frontal cortex. It's the frontal cortex which permits the anti-social aspects of the limbic drives to be realised in fantasies rather than acted out; it's the frontal cortex which channels raw sexual desires into socially acceptable paths of expression; and it's the frontal cortex which calibrates the potential benefit or damage of sexual and/or aggressive behaviour before either suppressing it or acting it out.

But the cortex is not simply the prim schoolmistress, slapping down the boisterous desires of the limbic system. It is every bit as much of a sexual organ itself. For if the limbic system is the seat of the raw and unharnessed sex drive, it is the cortex which is the seat of seduction. All the elaboration – and a large part of the pleasure – of sex originates there. And in a land where murdering one's competitors and raping one's conquests is forbidden, it's the cunning cortex which has developed an awesome array of sexual alternatives.

David Buss, whom we met earlier in the chapter while examining male fantasies, is also interested in the panoply of techniques men use to make them a reality. Where the brashest, boldest, brawniest, best-looking males had already corralled the largest number of the most fertile females, the rest of mankind had to live by wile. And they could direct it in two ways. First, by derogating other men and making them seem less attractive to women than they actually were; second, by exaggerating their own appeal.

In a study published in *The Journal of Sex Research* in 1994, Buss asked twenty-five male students what were the most effective ways for promoting sexual encounters. Derogation of competitors and the promotion of one's own attributes were both high on the list, with derogation tactics including 'putting down the insensitive behaviour of same-sex rivals' and self-promotion tactics including 'displaying strength . . . displaying status cues . . . and increasing perceived mate value through flirting with others'.

Careful deployment of designer logos; insouciant remarks about a rival's unattractive personality or lack of career success; hints dropped casually about telephone calls from other women; sudden enthusiasm to unscrew that unforgiving jam-jar top over breakfast the next morning – what man doesn't recognise the picture? Unprepared to outpunch their rivals, men are trying to outmanoeuvre them. And unwilling to seize their sexual partners, they attempt to seduce them.

Geoffrey Miller, one of the younger breed of evolutionary psychologists whose own cortex (framed by pre-Raphaelite curls) has wrestled with the question for years, even argues that this battle of sexual wits may be the reason the uniquely large human cortex developed in the first place. It's not a harness to keep the limbic system in check, he suggests, so much as a device 'to attract and retain mates'. The larger it became, the better it got at outwitting rivals and seducing partners, and the more partners that were seduced, the more frequently larger cortexes appeared in subsequent generations, creating an evolutionary arms race which resulted in the uniquely large brain-size of the modern human. Miller's thesis is not yet generally accepted, but one thing is certain: it is the cortex that has allowed the human mating system to become so elaborate and refined, giving us the words with which to woo, the songs with which to seduce, and the guile to make us plot, persist, and persuade. By a twist of fate, it's also the peculiar size of the cortex which has led to the third fundamental cornerstone of male sexual desire: a nod to monogamy.

A nod to monogamy

Consider the parable of the sower. Much of the seed which he strewed so generously by the wayside and in the verges never reached its full potential. On stony ground, or choked by thistles, or eaten by birds, the precious grain was unable to bring forth its harvest. Only the seed which fell on good ground was able to grow to maturity and reproduce in its turn. The same principle applies to human reproduction.

Three million years ago, when early man was roaming the grasslands of Africa, reproduction was considerably less costly than it is today. Hominid babies arrived in a more advanced state, able to start walking relatively soon after they were born. Before long, they could start feeding themselves, and from a very early age they were helping their group forage for food. But as the human brain began to grow, it needed a larger skull to contain it, and the larger the skull became, the more difficult it was for mothers to give birth. Walking upright demanded one form of female pelvis, but producing big-headed babies demanded another. A compromise had to be struck, because if a child got stuck in its mother's pelvis during delivery, it would mean certain death for both.

As a result, women began to give birth to their babies sooner, before their brains were fully developed. And while this had certain advantages for the child's future reproductive potential, it did little for his early survivability. Human babies are unique for their comparative helplessness at birth, spending the first year or so of their lives like external foetuses, relying on their mothers for every aspect of their well-being. This was the first problem created by large brains. But there was a second one, too: large brains needed a more protein-rich diet, and protein largely meant meat. Whereas early humans had previously subsisted on a predominantly vegetarian diet supplemented by occasional protein from animal kills, now they needed a much higher meat-to-vegetable ratio, and a mother whose mobility had been reduced by a dependent infant could not provide it alone.

It's at just about this point in human prehistory that men had to adapt to the fact that there was more to reproductive success than chasing round trying to mate with every fertile female in sight. A male who did this might beget more children, but his genes would never spread if none of them survived. And so it was that the male urge to philander had to be balanced with a completely different impulse: the impulse to stay around and help to provide for mother and infant.

It's probably too generous to suggest that men developed this urge naturally, or that they willingly became reliable partners and attentive fathers. As we will discover in the next chapter, women may well have been the driving force behind this move, developing a barrage of biological techniques to induce and enforce continued male attention. But whatever the precise sequence of events leading to what has become known as 'male parental investment', it is, for now, enough to recognise that the genes of men who stuck around and contributed to the welfare of their women and children were, on the whole, going to do better than those of men who did not. As a result, the genes (or psychological adaptations) for fatherhood would be likely to spread. The paternal devotion of the 'new man' is not just an expression of the sentimental

1990s *Zeitgeist*: it's every bit as much a primal male urge as the desire to sleep around.

But there was one rider to this new-found attentiveness. If a man was going to stay put, he needed to be sure that the children whose futures he was helping to assure were actually his. There would be no more fruitless waste of time and energy, genetically speaking, than to rear and protect another man's children as if they were his own. Thus, the male inclination to monogamy was driven by two necessities: first to promote the survival of the child, and second to guard the mother and make sure she was not open to impregnation by another man. How, though, could the two strategies for devoted attention and rampant philandering be reconciled?

For the despots of the ancient empires, it was easy. Hammurabi of Babylon, Akhenaten of Egypt, Fei-ti of China and all the others mentioned earlier in this chapter had enough power and sufficient cash to protect and provision for legions of women – and their children. They had no need to confine themselves to one, and no intention of doing so. The energy they displayed in amassing their harems was matched only by the cruelty with which they punished other men who infiltrated them. In the sixteenth century, a man caught dallying with one of the Aztec emperor Montezuma's concubines was to be 'stoned and thrown in the river or to buzzards', while anyone foolhardy enough to attempt a liaison with one of the Inca ruler's personal virgins could expect to be gathered up, along with his wife, children, relations, servants and all the inhabitants of his village, whereupon the whole party would be put to death, the village pulled to pieces and the site strewn with stones so that, as Inca historian Garcilaso de la Vega noted, 'the birthplace of so bad a son might remain for ever desolate and accursed'.

These techniques, of course, left the vast majority of less powerful, less successful men competing ever more desperately for an already depleted number of women. And in a world where permanent access to any woman at all came to be quite a prize, the best way to achieve it would be to promise lifelong investment both to her and to any children born from the union. This is the origin of monogamous marriage, the system we have inherited in the West to this day. In cultures where it has been forcibly policed, with powerful sanctions for all who stray, monogamy has been a reasonably effective tool in securing a good genetic deal for both sexes. Women have the guarantee of long-term investment from a single man;

and men have the guarantee that their investment is being channelled into their own genetic offspring.

By the most unlikely route, this is the system that now prevails on Pitcairn. After all the bloodshed, and having buried the other remaining man on the island, John Adams was plagued by a series of vivid and frightening dreams. All his sins were relived and his punishment appeared certain. Moved by his conscience and much preoccupied by the teachings of the single Bible left on the island, Adams threw his energies into turning Pitcairn into a model Christian community. Propped up by various missionaries over the succeeding two centuries, the Pitcairners of today are staunch Seventh-Day Adventists, attending church every Sunday, praying for the forgiveness of sins and joining themselves in holy, faithful, monogamous matrimony. When Donald Brown and Dana Hotra, two anthropologists from the University of California at Santa Barbara, decided to look at the Pitcairn records over those two hundred years, expecting them to show numerous signs of male attempts at cuckoldry and deception, they were amazed at how sexually faithful the islanders seem to have been. Perhaps when one considers how close-knit the community must have remained, with never more than a hundred members, it's less surprising. Any male attempts at philandering would soon have been stopped by other males fearful that this might leave them without a slice of the reproductive pie. And with the memory of such violence in their recent history, who would dare transgress?

In addition to despotic harem-building and faithful monogamy, there is a third possible response to the apparently conflicting male drives to invest in a wife and children, and to philander with as many women as possible. It's most common in cultures which uphold an ideal of monogamy, but which fail to enforce it upon men with any particular energy – contemporary European and American cultures, for example. In these societies, the most attractive male option, from a genetic point of view, is to marry a faithful, trustworthy wife whose unquestioned offspring one can legitimately supervise, and then to hunt for casual sex on the side.

David Buss goes so far as to argue that men may have developed a sort of internal calibrating system which files women according to whether they would make good wives or good one-night stands. As a result of a survey conducted in the early 1990s which asked men to specify what sort of qualities they sought in long-term mates compared to short-term ones, he found clear patterns emerging. For a start, most men require lower

standards of attractiveness when seeking one-night stands. They're willing
to accept a wider age range in their temporary partner, and lower levels
of such assets as charm, honesty, kindness, intelligence, wealth, sense of
humour, and emotional stability. The absolute negatives could be whittled
down to only two factors: low sex drive and hairiness.

The really interesting findings came later, when Buss found that the very
qualities which made women attractive as long-term partners made them
unattractive as short-term partners and vice versa. For example, on a scale
of importance from −3 (absolutely negative) to +3 (indispensable), men
rated 'need and willingness for commitment' as a tremendously positive
+2.17 in a long-term or marriage partner, but a definitely undesirable
−1.4 in a short-term or temporary partner. By contrast, sexual availability,
sexual experience, and sexual promiscuity were abhorred in long-term
partners, but positively sought-after in short-term partners. As Mae West
said, 'Men like women with a past because they hope history will repeat
itself.'

Elizabeth Hill, mounting an experiment in the mid-1980s, illustrated
this see-saw effect graphically. Men were exposed to slides of female models wearing clothes which got progressively tighter and more revealing.
She wasn't surprised to discover that the skimpier the clothes became,
the more attractive men found their wearers as possible dating partners or
sex partners, but the less attractive as marriage partners. We're back with
Robert Trivers: the more a man will be expected to invest in any possible
offspring, the choosier he will be. The time-honoured mother's advice that
a daughter should hold on to her virtue if she wishes to make a good
marriage may have a sound, if depressing, basis in evolutionary logic.

We started this tale in a land without laws, hoping to find the natural
pattern of male sexual desire. But instead of one man living with one wife
in a settled peaceable Utopia, we found bitter and deadly struggles in
which men competed and murdered for access to women. Seeking an
explanation, the question of human evolutionary design was examined.
What are we made for, we asked, and the answer came back: sex. In men,
this meant fighting for access to women, then mating with the largest
possible number, a pattern that was repeated with unfailing regularity by
male leaders, whose lives were not subject to the restraints they placed
on their subjects. Yet it appears that the only thing unique about these
men was their power to realise in life what the rest of their male subjects
could only dream of. For when we looked inside the minds of all men,

we identified a number of programmes designed to make them both relish competition and savour the prospect of sex with lots of women. These appear to be wired into the very fabric of their bodies, from the hormones which circulate in their blood, to the structure and function of the different parts of their brains. Even the drive to monogamy, which developed as an unforeseen side effect of a sexually effective cortex (one which was masterful at slander and seduction), turns out to be nothing more than a cynical attempt to have one's cake and eat it.

It's a bleak picture for those who cling, Rousseau-like, to the belief that humans are naturally good, and even bleaker for those who believe that men and women have been put on this Earth to serve and support each other. But we've only had half the picture. For the purposes of clarity, I've considered the basic sexual instincts of the male in isolation from those of the female. In reality, of course, none of these could have evolved without women's participation, influence and response at every stage. So if the picture thus far seems to imply that women have been little more than passive spectators of their own sexual fate, collected by the powerful, wooed by the weak, and exploited by all, read on. For the next chapter is all about the basic sexual instincts of the human female and, as we'll discover, passivity and inertia have never entered into it.

2

Women

Peter Hegedus was the first to go, poisoned by his wife in his sleep. The year was 1914; the place, the little village of Nagyrev, some sixty miles south-east of Budapest on the river Tisza. The Austro-Hungarian empire was under threat from the Russians, and the First World War had begun. Like men from all over the hinterlands of Eastern Europe, the husbands and fiancés of the young women in Nagyrev were being called up to fight, and one by one, they were leaving. Some departed with tears and farewells; others slipped away silently, in the small hours before dawn.

We can only speculate on how the womenfolk felt at this sudden absence. Some, no doubt, were heartbroken. Others, lonely and afraid. Some, perhaps, relieved. All we know for sure is that things were soon to change in Nagyrev.

Slowly, without their men, the women were forced to become more independent, taking on sole responsibility for their homes, their children and their own lives. Many began taking an active part in the running of the village; others entered local government. Gradually, over the next few months, a sense of optimism, even good cheer, returned to the village. Then, with some excitement, it was announced that a prisoner of war camp was to be constructed a few hundred yards down the road. It took only a matter of weeks to build, and it would hold many hundreds of captives. A whisper went round the houses. What would these young men be like? Would they be safely confined? Were they dangerous? It did not take long to find out. Over the ensuing weeks, nearly every one of the young women of Nagyrev had made contact with the camp and selected a lover. Then the older women followed suit, also taking lovers. Some became dissatisfied with only a single man, and gradually, enjoying two or three became the norm. Each woman built up her own supply, having sex with whoever she wished whenever she wished. Even if the men had been tempted to complain, they couldn't. They were prisoners of war and had little option but to obey.

This situation persisted until wounded and war-weary husbands started returning from the Front. The reception they received was extremely cool. The women of Nagyrev had experienced a taste of sexual independence and real power, and were now disinclined to give it up. So disinclined, in fact, that they turned to the local midwife, Mrs Fazekas, for help. Mrs Fazekas was an opportunist who had discovered a way to make poison by boiling the glue off the back of conscription posters. For a small price, she dispensed the deadly cocktails to her female clients, and the murders began in earnest; over one hundred in all between 1914 and 1929.

This bizarre episode might have gone completely undiscovered were it not for a Mrs Ladislaus Szabo, who failed to prescribe the correct dosage to a man she 'disliked' and who was accused of having tried to poison his wine. Reluctant to face the music alone, she implicated her friend Mrs Bukenowski, who confessed that she had received a supply of arsenic from Mrs Fazekas. Mrs Fazekas denied everything but was trailed by police as she returned home, stopping on the way at numerous houses to warn her clients that the game might be up. The police arrested a woman in every house that she entered and finally seized her as she stepped inside her own front door, where pots of soaking flypapers incriminated her without the need for a confession. All in all, twenty-six women were brought to trial. Eight were sentenced to death, seven to life imprisonment, and the rest to varying terms in jail.

Though many of the murderesses had killed lovers as well as husbands, it was the spousal homicides which formed the clearest and most persistent pattern. When asked why they had done it, Rosalie Sebestyen and Rosa Hoyba answered simply that they found their husbands 'boring', while Mrs Juliane Lipka told of her advice to a neighbour whose marriage was on the rocks: 'I was sorry for the wretched woman, so I gave her a bottle of poison and told her that if nothing else helped . . . try that.'

Although the story of 'The Angel-Makers of Nagyrev', as they became known, is true, it reads more like a parable. What would happen if women openly held sway over men; if they could enjoy and dispose of them as they wished without fear of punishment or retribution? What if all the established men were removed from the equation, together with their capacity to punish or provide, and a new consignment of powerless males introduced with whom the women were free to do as they pleased? In these circumstances, would women pursue a course of rampant philandering, picking up and putting down whichever men took their fancy, or would they sit demurely at home, uninterested in the possibilities of casual sex and waiting patiently for their husbands to return? At the time when the events at Nagyrev were unfolding, this was not an idle guessing game. It was a burning question, for the twentieth century had dawned with ignorance and anxiety about the true pattern of female sexuality. For many years, the issue had been hotly debated by two extremely partisan camps.

A dark continent

On the one hand were those who held that women were every bit as sexually voracious and variety-seeking as men. This we might term the 'active' camp, and its supporters had a long, distinguished and international pedigree, stretching from the Indian sage Vatsyayana, who wrote in the *Kama Sutra* that, 'When women cannot come on to a man, they even fall lustfully on one another, for they will never be true to their husbands,' to the medieval European witch-hunters Jakob Sprenger and Heinrich Krämer, whose *Malleus Maleficarum* depicts women as 'beautiful to look upon, contaminating to the touch, and deadly to keep'. They believed that 'all witchcraft comes from carnal lust, which in women is insatiable'.

In radical opposition, the second body of thought held that women, if they had a sex drive at all, would keep it well hidden and infrequently indulged. This we might term the 'passive' model, and it reached its apogee in Victorian England, when the eminent surgeon Dr William Acton announced that 'the majority of women, happily for them, are not much troubled by sexual feelings of any kind'. He didn't deny that some women were capable of being aroused, but he suggested that they were 'sad exceptions', and on a fast track to a 'form of insanity that those who visit lunatic asylums must be fully conversant with'.

It seemed that the debate would never be settled. Most obviously, the definitive evidence could simply never be found. Setting aside the extra-ordinary circumstances at Nagyrev, women had never enjoyed sufficient power or freedom to express their sexuality without male coercion or control. Throughout history and across the world, men had always had the lion's share of property, money, freedom, physical strength and political power. No culture had yet been found where women were entirely free to make their own choices.

A second problem, as with most matters sexual, was that almost all of the theorising was being done by men, whose views tended to reveal more about male hopes and fears concerning female sexuality than about female sexuality itself. Women untroubled by sexual feelings were likely to make good wives and dependable mothers, while those filled with lust might always be open to bouts of commitment-free copulation.

Still a third problem was that even when the best minds had struggled with the task as objectively as they could, their results remained filled with uncertainties and contradictions. The pioneering nineteenth- and early-twentieth-century sexologists like Richard von Krafft-Ebing, Magnus Hirschfeld and Henry Havelock Ellis appeared to take first one position and then the other. Krafft-Ebing's epic investigation into sexual pathology, *Psychopathia Sexualis*, comments on 'so many husbands' confidential complaints to the doctor of the frigidity of their wives', yet also contains lengthy sections on nymphomania. And while some of Ellis's case studies read like a litany in female anorgasmia, his writings overall suggested that women could and did take pleasure in sex.

Perhaps these seeming contradictions explain why, in Western history at least, men often chose to believe in both images at once, either dividing women in general into two distinct groups, the 'madonnas' whom they married and the 'whores' they would visit on the side; or, rather improbably, dividing individual women into two separate sections, meeting in the middle. 'Down from the waist they are centaurs,' cried Shakespeare's King Lear, 'though women all above.' Magnus Hirschfeld even made a fanciful attempt to reconcile the two camps with his theory that female arousal lay dormant until awakened by a substance found in male sperm called 'andrin', which allowed it to blossom and grow.

Rumblings of discontent at these reductive, male-oriented and often rather Gothic views began to be heard by the turn of the century, when women started battling to become physicians and writers themselves; but for decades, efforts to popularise contraception and allow women to take more control over their lives were a more urgent priority than investigating the female sex drive. Indeed, some early feminists wished to play down the sexuality issue or avoid it altogether, feeling that too much emphasis on pleasure might prejudice their cause. 'Votes for women and chastity for men' was one of the favourite slogans of the English suffragette movement.

By the time feminist thought really took hold in the West during the 1960s and 1970s, the task of investigating female sexuality with at least some input from a female perspective could no longer be ignored. In 1966, husband-and-wife team William Masters and Virginia Johnson collaborated on a detailed examination of female sexuality, whose results were published in their book *Human Sexual Response*. Here, aided by a panoply of electric probes and monitors, they were able to provide the following hyper-real though uniquely unerotic account of the female orgasm:

> Strong muscle contractions started in the outer third of the vaginal barrel, with the first contraction lasting from two to four seconds and later contractions occurring at 0.8-second intervals; slight expansion of the inner two-thirds of the vagina; contraction of the uterus; peak intensity and distribution of the sex flush; frequently strong muscular contractions in many parts of the body; possibly doubling of the respiratory rate and heart rate; blood pressure elevation to as much as a third above normal; and vocalization in some instances.

Acton, and all who still gathered round his banner, would have been horrified. Not only was this living, detailed proof of female arousability, it was collected during an episode of masturbation, which he would scarcely have acknowledged as a possibility, let alone a pleasurable activity. And as if to rub salt into the wound, surveys quickly followed which suggested that at least 50 per cent of women experienced orgasm regularly; that it was most easily achieved as a result of clitoral stimulation; that it generally took longer to achieve than male orgasm, but that once attained, it could last longer and be repeated more swiftly. What's more, intercourse was not necessary for the female orgasm to occur. As Shere Hite documented in her 1976 survey, *The Hite Report on Female Sexuality*, penile penetration was actually a much less effective way to achieve it than masturbation.

For any who still held doubts, here was living proof that some women, at least, could and did take pleasure in sex and that they didn't need to rely on their husbands to provide it. But the 'active' versus 'passive' debate had not ended. It was just gearing up for another round, as partisans in each camp modified their positions, conceded a few points to the opposition, then sharpened their pencils for the next big clash. Moving away from the existence of the female orgasm, they turned instead to its function. What was it actually for?

In the West, there had traditionally been two answers to this question, both dating from the time of the ancient Greeks. The first was that female orgasm somehow aided conception, with the shuddering contractions that signalled its arrival helping to waft sperm to their ultimate destination. The other was that orgasm was good for a woman's overall health.

It was a version of the latter idea that was picked up and advocated by the feminist psychiatrist Mary Jane Sherfey, in her controversial 1972 publication *The Nature and Evolution of Female Sexuality*. Here, Sherfey painted a picture of our earliest ancestors as living in groups ruled by sexually promiscuous females, who copulated wildly and frequently with whichever males they selected, with orgasm helping to remove unwanted 'venous congestion' from their pelvic regions. Evolution, she suggested, would have favoured women who were motivated to engage in sex often, and who were capable of having lengthy, powerful and frequent orgasms. This apparently idyllic matriarchal society, with everyone happily accepting the 'rule of the mother', had been a favourite fantasy of radical feminists as early as the nineteenth century. Unfortunately, the societal model which Sherfey advanced found little support from archaeology, and her theory of the female orgasm had no basis in modern medicine. As a result, her views never caught on with the scientists, but they inspired feminist thinkers from other disciplines to provide more plausible scenarios.

Chief among these was Sarah Hrdy, a primatologist of Czech descent, much of whose fieldwork has been conducted in India, among a species of old-world monkey called the Hanuman langur. Observing these animals in the wild, Hrdy noticed two significant facts. First, the females (in common with several other species of primate) showed signs of an assertive and active sexuality. And second, whenever new males moved into the group, they would attempt to seize and kill its suckling infants. The reason for the infanticide was brutally clear. By killing a female's young, a newly arrived male could bring its mother back on heat and mate with her himself.

In such a ruthless environment, females needed cunning strategies to foil the killers. Perhaps, reasoned Hrdy, the females had developed an active sexuality in order to seek out large numbers of males and mate with them, thus confusing each as to whether or not he was the father of any new children. With the ever-present possibility that any of them might be, the best-case scenario was that they would help feed and protect both mother and infant; the worst-case scenario was that they would leave them alone. In either case, murder would be forestalled. Thus, in Hrdy's re-creation of what may have been our own distant primate past, an active sexuality among females was both a tool for extracting resources for men, and a shield for protecting children. And if the urge to seek sex with a variety of partners continued to evoke at least one of these benefits, it made perfect sense for a proactive female sexuality to have clung on through evolutionary time.

So much for the modified 'active' camp. But the majority of evolutionary thinkers take another tack. Women do indeed take pleasure in sex, they say, but it's a daintier, more disinterested pleasure, revolving chiefly around social and emotional interaction. It's essentially the old 'passive' position, with a few added orgasms. One of the most influential among the new 'passivists' was the aforementioned Donald Symons. Then a young anthropologist at the University of Santa Barbara, Symons argued that there could be little specific reason for women to have a powerful sex drive, or indeed a clitoris to fuel it, because 'it is difficult to see how expending time and energy pursuing the will-o'-the-wisp of sexual satiation, endlessly and fruitlessly attempting to make a bottomless cup flow over, could conceivably contribute to a female's reproductive success'. Whatever the ancient Greeks may have thought, orgasm was certainly not necessary for conception; it was definitely not automatically obtained by vaginal intercourse; the venous congestion idea had been debunked; and the theory that women were sexually insatiable in order to promote the survival of their offspring seemed to Symons both maladroit and misinformed. Indeed, he argued, 'Insatiability would markedly interfere with the adaptively significant activities of food-gathering and childcare.' Symons didn't deny that the female orgasm existed, or that women could and did find pleasure in sex. But for him, all this was a by-product of the evolutionary process. Active sexuality was useful in men, so there might be vestiges of it in women. But these vestiges were not specifically shaped by evolution.

Active or passive? Insatiable or coy? The debate continued through the

1970s and early '80s, with further contributions from primatologists, anthropologists, even ornithologists. Then, with a spate of new behavioural studies on the sexual psychology of the human male, certain experimenters started to apply their techniques to the female as well.

Quality not quantity

In the last chapter, I mentioned three contemporary biologists who have played a key role in expanding our understanding of the evolutionary forces which underpin all life: John Maynard Smith, George Williams and Robert Trivers. It is the last of these whose work is most directly responsible for allowing us to make predictions about the sexual natures of men and women, and then to test them.

Trivers's theory about the different levels of investment required from males and females in the fertilisation, gestation and rearing of their offspring suggested that whichever sex bore the heaviest burden would be the more careful chooser. In the case of humans, men often invest unusually highly, helping their partners through pregnancy and supporting their children for many years after birth. But, as we've seen, this is not always the case. In fact, for most of our evolutionary history, the best way for a man to increase his overall reproductive success may have been to invest in a few carefully supervised, legitimate children, while pursuing a course of rampant philandering on the side. This is possible because men have the option of investing nothing more in their offspring than a few minutes of mating time and a small package of cheaply produced, easily replenished sperm.

This is not an option open to women. First, women produce far fewer egg cells than men. Second, each one has to be loaded with nutrients to help a new foetus on its way. Third, each successful fertilisation ushers in a draining and burdensome nine-month period of pregnancy, during which the foetus relies on its mother for every aspect of its continued survival. The mother feeds the foetus internally, protects it physically, and maintains a round-the-clock vigil on behalf of its health by increasing her sensitivity to toxins (one of the origins of morning sickness). Finally, when the child is born, it is the mother who continues to provide the major source of nourishment: milk. The average mother lactates for months after the child is born, which tends temporarily to suppress her capacity to ovulate and bear further children. Taken together, these factors mean that, for every successful fertilisation, the minimum level of investment required from a woman is enormous.

Today, of course, the advent of birth control means that women need not anticipate the burdens of pregnancy every time they have sex. For the first time in our history, sex is not inexorably linked to reproduction. But for the vast majority of our evolutionary past, if a woman made a single lapse with the wrong man the possibility of several wasted years loomed. As a result, we might reasonably expect women to show less concern about the quantity of their partners and more about their quality.

So what kind of mental mechanisms might have evolved to shape the female sex drive? Let's return to the campus and find out. When considering the male sex drive, we looked at a number of studies showing that men are programmed to want sex with a wide variety of potentially fertile women. As we saw in Russell Clark and Elaine Hatfield's experiment, male passers-by propositioned by a group of attractive female college students became more and more enthusiastic the more directly sexual the offers became. Fifty per cent agreed to a date, 69 per cent agreed to go back to the woman's apartment, and 75 per cent consented to immediate sex. But this wasn't the end of the story.

What Clark and Hatfield had tried on men, they now tried on women too, asking male students to position themselves around the campus and ask the same questions of female passers-by. They were careful to ensure that the male students were neatly turned out and that they would seem as unthreatening as possible. The results were extremely clear-cut. While approximately half the women agreed to go on a date (the same as for the men), the numbers plummeted for anything more immediate or suggestive. Only 6 per cent of those asked agreed to go back to the male student's apartment, and none at all consented to immediate sex. Furthermore, when Clark and Hatfield looked at the nature of the negative responses made by both sexes, they found an even clearer divide, with men much more likely to express regret, and women much more likely to express scorn. 'I can't tonight, but tomorrow would be fine' was a typical response from a man, while 'you've got to be kidding' was more characteristic of the women.

Clark and Hatfield are careful to point out that an evolutionary explanation is not the only one that can be offered here. Women may have been more reluctant because traditionally they have been conditioned to refuse such offers. And whatever precautions had been taken to make the men seem unthreatening, some might still have been cautious about the dangers of being alone with a total stranger. Other researchers, however, have been much more detailed in their investigations, and much more forthright in their conclusions.

One of these is David Buss, who in the early 1990s questioned 148 men and women about how long they felt they would need to have known someone before they had intercourse with them, assuming that they found the person in question desirable. After they had known a potential sex partner for five years, both men and women stated that they would probably have intercourse with them, but at every time interval briefer than five years, the women were less likely to consent to sex than men. When it came down to one week, men were still, on average, positive about the idea of sex, but women were pretty negative; after both had known the other for only an hour, men were only slightly disinclined to have sex, whereas women considered it a virtual impossibility.

Buss then asked the same men and women how many sexual partners they would ideally like to have over a series of given time intervals; for example, within the next month, the next year, the next five years, the next ten years and, finally, over their entire lifetime. At each interval, he found that women expressed a desire for fewer partners, wanting on average no more than one over the next year, no more than two over the next five years, and no more than four or five over their entire lifetime. Men, on the other hand, wanted at least six over the next year and, on average, more than eighteen over their entire lifetime.

While there was considerable variability from individual to individual, as there must be from one type of study group to another, Buss took the unanimous overall direction of these results to indicate that women must have an underlying sexual psychology, formed through evolution, which encourages them to be less interested than men in the number and variety of people with whom they wish to have sex. But if they're less concerned by quantity, what about quality? Do women seek higher standards in those with whom they consent to have sex, or does the lot simply fall to whoever passes when they happen to be in the mood?

To examine this question, Douglas Kenrick and his colleagues assembled a list of twenty-four positive characteristics – including kindness, intelligence, earning capacity, physical attractiveness, friendliness and creativity – and asked both men and women what would be the minimum percentage of each quality they would require in a partner before agreeing to date them, have sex with them, steady-date them, or marry them. In each type of relationship, the women demanded higher percentages of almost every quality than the men, but the most marked difference was at the level of casual sex, where women demanded that a man score an overall average of at least 46 per cent, while men demanded only about 35 per cent.

David Buss picked up on Kenrick's study and took it one stage further, seeking to elucidate how men and women reacted to negative as well as to positive qualities in potential mates. With his students, he assembled a list of sixty-one characteristics which might be unappealing to either sex. These included 'unaffectionate', 'bigoted', 'boring', 'cheap', 'dishonest', 'dumb', 'lacks ambition', 'has bad breath' and so on. He then asked men and women to rate these on a scale which ranged from 'extremely desirable' to 'extremely undesirable'. As expected, with over three-quarters of the characteristics, women expressed higher exclusionary standards than men, displaying a particular concern over those who were 'mentally abusive, physically abusive, bisexual, disliked by others, drank a lot of alcohol, dumb, uneducated, a gambler, old, possessive, promiscuous, self-centred, selfish, lacking a sense of humour, not sensual, short, submissive, violent, and wimpy'. It is a testament not just to female quality control but also to male urgency that the men considered these characteristics undesirable but often not prohibitive.

Overall, then, Trivers's theory that the sex which invests most in its offspring is likely to be the sex which chooses its partners more carefully seems to be holding up. According to evolutionary psychologists at least, women are less likely to seek sex out, less likely to accept offers from those who proposition them, and especially reluctant to jump into bed with those they have known for only a matter of minutes. The majority require relatively high standards of acceptability from their potential partners, and they apply higher exclusionary criteria. But does this really mean that women are less sexual than men, or simply that they are sexually different? To answer this question, we need to leave the campus and enter the laboratory.

The Sex Chair

The Sex Chair resembles something from an early *Thunderbirds* episode. With levers on the arm-rests, buttons on the table in front, and wires trailing from underneath the seat, it is a fully automated arousal detector, designed to measure the sexual responses of whoever sits in it. Some of the equipment is designed to register conscious arousal. For instance, there's a lever which the subject manipulates to indicate his or her psychological reaction to stimuli he or she is shown. But some of the array of instruments are also designed to recognise smaller, often unnoticed, signals occurring within the body. Chief among these is what is known as a 'vaginal plethysmograph', a sort of genital lie-detector which fits inside the vagina and picks up even the smallest variations in genital response: a slight swelling of labial tissue, or the beginnings of vaginal engorgement.

The Chair is owned by the University of Amsterdam, and one of its chief operators is Dr Ellen Laan, whose ingenious investigations into the complexities of female desire are making her one of the hottest (as well as one of the youngest) names in current sex research.

Laan thought that the debate over whether women are inherently more or less sexual than men was deeply flawed by the questions which were being asked. Most tests tended to put them in situations where men would respond sexually, find their response was less immediate, and conclude that women were less arousable. But she was sure that these results had less to do with the nature of female sexuality than with the nature of the stimuli. To get a more nuanced picture, the stimuli had to be more carefully chosen. Laan decided to use the chair to measure the levels of arousal experienced by various women in response to two kinds of pornographic film: one made by a male director for a male-oriented market, and another made by a female director with female arousal in mind. If female sexuality was inherently different from its male counterpart, she reasoned, these two styles of film might give her a reading on whether it differed simply in degree or, more subtly, in kind.

The choice of male-oriented film was determined by the highest lending rate in Laan's local video store. It was enacted in what she describes as 'an obvious brothel-like environment, in which the man was awaiting the services of an unacquainted woman . . . there was no foreplay at all, and non-sexual details were minimised'. The female-oriented film, on the other hand, made by an ex-porn star dissatisfied with the male bias in pornography, was set in an elevator in which mutual attraction developed between two people 'resulting in stroking, kissing, and eventually in mutual undressing'.

Laan put nearly fifty subjects in the chair, of differing ages, personalities, and religious convictions. The films were run one after the other, and slowly the results began to emerge. First, as Laan had expected, there was considerable variation between the women, with those who had not previously experienced pornography reporting less arousal than those who were more familiar with it; and with older women showing less genital (though no less psychological) arousal to both types of stimulus. Yet despite these individual differences, there were several clear overall trends which were as surprising as they were suggestive.

The first was that the levels of genital arousal picked up by the plethysmograph were very high, and generally just as high in response to both styles of film. On a genital level at least, women were responding positively to quick, anonymous bouts of sex. But when Laan turned to the results shown by the lever, a very different pattern emerged. Here, the women indicated that they had consistently felt much more psychologically aroused by the female film than by the male one, with the adjectives they used to describe the former including 'exciting, sensual, cute, arousing, better, real and surprising' with 'awful, coarse, ludicrous, banal, distasteful, obscene, and unaesthetic' characterising their response to the latter.

The clear disjunction between genital arousal and psychological arousal raised very interesting questions. Physiological measurement was simply not telling the whole story. In the case of males, where the penis was a straightforward, accurate, and highly visible gauge of arousal, recording its changes was a straightforward and reasonable method of assessment. But Laan's results suggested that in female arousal, the brain was playing a much more important and much more independent role. Could it be possible that it required certain criteria to be met before allowing its owner to recognise arousal and respond to the signals that her genitals had begun to show? This new scenario seemed to make most previous models of female sexuality rather simplistic. Debates about its active or passive nature may have been missing the point. Most intriguing, now, was the complex interplay of psychological and physical arousal. It was clear that psychological arousal was a highly important, primary factor in female desire for sex; even more important, perhaps, than sheer physical genital arousal. But what conditions would best create it?

Mr Right

It's half-past eleven in a busy corporate office. Well-groomed executives sit at their desks, sifting through the morning's mail, tapping on their computers, and making assignments on the telephone. Everything seems cool, calm, and collected. Then, suddenly, no one seems to be doing any work. A ripple goes around the office. The executives whisper to each other, with sly grins and a hefty dose of innuendo. Everybody's rushing to the window and craning to catch a glimpse of well-toned, tanned and exposed flesh. As the object of their desire opens a canned drink and thirstily consumes it, the audience at the window sighs wistfully. Their eyes follow every curve of this gorgeous creature's body. The sexual tension is simmering.

The catch, of course, is that in this highly successful television commercial, the highly-paid professional lechers are women, while the figure being lusted after is a muscular construction worker, stripped to the waist and enjoying his Diet Coke break. The commercial reverses all the usual visual clichés of sexy Californian girls caressing cans of sugary water, and reflects a new world where women earn their own living and choose their own partners. Some objected that it was just a new twist on an old theme; others that it was risibly out of touch with the real world, where construction workers are still usually the ones harassing the women. But the ad was a hit; perhaps because it tapped into an aspect of sexual desire which was just beginning to make itself felt in the global marketplace. The women in this ad know very little about their idol, and what they do know is not all positive. He seems to be diligent enough, but he's working on a building site, so he's unlikely to be rolling in money. They don't know where he's come from, what he's like, or where he's going. Basically, they've got little more to judge him on than his looks . . . and they're all entranced.

Women find handsome men attractive, even when they know nothing about them. This may sound like stating the obvious, but it bears repeating because, although it's demonstrably true in real life, it's a fact that evolutionary thinkers and scientists have traditionally tended to treat rather superficially.

Handsome men will pass their physical advantages down to the children of whoever they mate with, giving those children a head-start in the race for reproductive success. As we'll see later, the indices of conventional male good looks – a rugged jaw, broad shoulders, a full head of hair and a healthy physique – are also indications of genetic health and strength. Yet looks in the opposite sex seem to be less important to women than they are to men, and less important than other factors. In Douglas Kenrick's study of the percentages required of potential partners before women would consent to dating, having sex, steady dating or marrying them, 'good looks' was the only criterion where women, across the board, were ready to accept a lower percentage value than men. They were even prepared to consider men of below-average physical attractiveness . . . as long as they had other things to offer.

Legend has it that, some years ago, the actor Dustin Hoffman was sitting in a restaurant quietly enjoying dinner when he began to notice the attentions of a number of female diners. They were looking at him, whispering, giggling. Hoffman began to feel a little uncomfortable. Eventually, they approached him and asked for his autograph. One even asked him out on a date. At this point, Hoffman began to grow exasperated and, turning to his audience, uttered in mock dismay: 'Girls, please, where were you when I needed you?'

Hoffman is, by most standards, not conventionally handsome. As a male model, stripped to the waist and lined up next to the Diet Coke hunk, he probably wouldn't have made the grade. But Hoffman, like most famous men, has other attributes. In Glenn Wilson's study of British sexual fantasies, men were found to fantasise more frequently about group sex than any of the other scenarios he presented to them. But women had a very different fantasy life. For them, by far the most characteristic fantasy was straight, monogamous sex with a famous personality. The argument runs that famous men today, like village headmen in the past, and successful hunters during the early period in which we evolved, would have acquired the status and resources to furnish a woman and her children with more food and protection than the next man. Over the incremental advances of time, evolution would therefore have favoured women who developed mental programmes which allowed them to judge the signs of status within their particular environment and culture, and calibrate their desire accordingly.

Fame is not the only indicator of a man who is high in status and rich in resources. In 1986, the American psychologist Elizabeth Hill published the results of an experiment in which she asked her students to describe what sort of clothes they considered high-status men to wear, and what sort of clothes they considered low-status men to wear. Among the former were smart suits, polo shirts, designer jeans and expensive watches; among the latter were nondescript jeans, tank tops and T-shirts. She then photographed a number of different men in variations of both styles of dress and showed the photographs to a different group of female students, asking them to rate each one for attractiveness. Overall, the same models were found more attractive when wearing the high-status costumes than when wearing the low-status ones.

It's important to note, though, that it's not just status symbols, and the resources they indicate, that women find attractive. It's also those personality characteristics which indicate the capacity to acquire such symbols in the future. In most cultures, women rarely have the luxury of being able to wait for a man to achieve all that he sets out to do before pairing up with him; as a result they have to calibrate his desirability partly on unrealised potential.

To find out what these characteristics of future success might be, and to see how they correlated with female desire, psychologist Michael Wiederman examined more than a thousand personal ads placed in various American periodicals between January and June 1992. He speculated that, in an arena where men and women were paying to attract potential mates, they would be more than usually forthright in specifying the attributes they sought, and more than usually direct in how they expressed their priorities. Taking the various descriptions of what people wanted, and arranging them into categories, Wiederman noticed that terms indicating high status and plentiful resources (terms such as 'business owner', 'enjoys the finer things', 'successful', 'wealthy', 'well-to-do', and 'financially affluent') cropped up ten times as often in the women's wish lists as in the men's. But there was also a considerable female preference for terms like 'ambitious', 'industrious', 'career-oriented', and 'college-educated'; in other words, for terms which clearly indicated the potential to acquire status and amass resources in the future.

Wiederman's results have been backed up by numerous other studies covering different decades and geographical areas. The American periodical *The Journal of Home Economics* took the sexual temperature of the nation's youth in the 1940s, '50s and '60s and found in each decade that young women rated financial prospects as highly desirable (though not absolutely essential) in men they were considering dating. Douglas Kenrick, in his study of how intelligent, attractive and so on men and women had to be before they were considered sexually attractive by the opposite sex, found that earning capacity was much more important to women than to men; and David Buss, in a massive study of mating habits which covered ten thousand people in thirty-seven cultures around the world, found that women rated financial resources on average at least twice as highly as men did.

Some researchers argue that an evolutionary explanation is not justified here. Women only desire wealthy men, they say, because most cultures don't allow women to make much money for themselves. But the female preference for wealth seems to exist regardless of the financial status of the women in question. There is an unprecedented number of independent, self-supporting women with resources of their own in the world today, yet their mate preferences still seem to be following the age-old, evolved pattern of looking for men who can offer more. One study of American newly-wed couples in 1993 found that financially successful brides placed an even greater importance on their husbands' earning capacities than those who were less well-off. And another, conducted among female college students, reported that those who were likely to earn more in respected professions placed greater importance on the financial prospects of their potential husbands than those who were likely to earn less. Buss's fellow psychologist Bruce Ellis summed up the prospect for future mate choice by saying, 'Women's sexual tastes become more, rather than less, discriminatory as their wealth, power, and social status increase.'

The guarantee of satisfaction

Two factors then, are key in female mate selection. Good looks (which roughly translate as 'good genes'), and the capacity to acquire status and resources. But, looked at from an evolutionary point of view, there should be a third essential component to female desire. To discover what it is, we must travel to the town of Don Mills, Ontario, for this is the headquarters of Harlequin Enterprises, the world's most successful publisher of the product through which female fantasy finds its widest and most profitable expression: romantic fiction. Driven by purely commercial imperatives, the company has a clear remit to appeal to the largest possible number of consumers, and there is a constant feedback mechanism. The signal something's really hit the button is that it sells.

Harlequin was founded in Winnipeg by printing executive Richard Bonnycastle to meet the growing demand for paperback books in post-war Canada. At first, they published a wide range of genres, including Westerns, thrillers, craft books and classics, featuring such authors as Agatha Christie, Jean Plaidy, James Hadley Chase and Somerset Maugham. But also included in the list were a number of romances originally published by the British company Mills & Boon. It was Mary Bonnycastle, wife of the founder, who first noticed the popularity of what she called those 'nice little books with happy endings', and suggested that Harlequin should concentrate on selling them.

Fifty years later the company is in buoyant mood. It acquired Mills & Boon in the early 1970s, snapped up its major competitor, Silhouette, in 1984, and now has a 20 per cent share of the total global market in popular fiction, selling over two hundred million books a year to over fifty million readers in more than a hundred countries around the world. The books themselves come in several styles, from the 'gentle, tender love stories' of Harlequin Romance to the 'provocative, sensuous, passionate stories' of the Temptation series. Yet despite their surface variety, each is informed by the same editorial principle. The heroes are universally handsome, adventurous, and accompanied by what Harlequin editors call 'the guarantee of satisfaction'. This guarantee, though usually hidden at the outset, stipulates that the hero will ultimately fall in love with the heroine and show every sign of being prepared to live with her in a state of lifelong happiness, providing her and their children with the benefit of his long-term and exclusive care. In the more traditional imprints, a trip to the altar will almost certainly take place. In the racier novels, children are sometimes already on the way.

Rita Clay Estrada's *The Stormchaser*, a recent best-seller from the Temptation series, gives us the entire recipe in spades. In many ways, the story is startlingly modern. The characters live in a world where unhappy childhoods, failed marriages, long working days and personal insecurity abound. They work on personal computers, eat junk food, and have clearly recognisable flaws (the hero drinks beer from a can, the heroine worries about her stretchmarks). Yet the innovations only throw the eternal essentials into sharper relief.

Cane Mitchell, the handsome thirtysomething hero, follows in the wake of natural disasters, working as an insurance adjuster. Investigating a claim, he meets Bernadette Conrad, a widow with an eighteen-year-old son of her own, whose house has been destroyed in an earthquake. Their instant mutual attraction is frustrated by differences in class and career, but most of all by Cane's reluctance to consider a serious relationship after the break-up of his marriage and a string of short-term girlfriends. Nevertheless, they kiss and make love soon after they meet and, for a blissful interlude, they move into temporary accommodation together. Unfortunately, given their conflicting goals, it cannot last. Bernadette wants a lasting and deeply-rooted commitment that Cane is unwilling to give; they break up in a welter of tears and confusion. But there is a further, complicating factor. Unbeknown to Cane, Bernadette is pregnant with his child, conceived accidentally. Facing up to the future, she decides to go it alone and have the baby regardless. He, meanwhile, suffers agonies of separation and regret – and finally dares to attempt a reconciliation. Over the final pages, the denouement plays itself out in three distinct stages.

First, Cane announces that he is deeply in love with Bernadette:

> Cane stood and faced her, letting the blanket drop to the concrete. His expression was heartbreakingly filled with love. 'No. I know what I want, and it's right here in front of me. Forever.'

After this, an oblique marriage proposal heralds his intention to look after her permanently:

> 'And do you want a formal wedding or can we elope?'
> Her solemn expression turned into a broad grin. 'A formal wedding, a big one.'
> 'Damn,' he muttered. 'I had a feeling you'd say that.'

Finally, Cane is faced with the first test of his promised permanent care, a child to look after as well as a wife.

> Taking a deep breath, she moved her hands down to her abdomen, cradling the slight roundness there. 'Hurricane Mitchell, if you run from me now, know that you'll be running from two of us. There will be no third chance for either one. We either commit to be together

and raise this child with all the love and caring we all deserve, or we call it off now, while I can still function without you.'

'Hurricane' rises to the task, and the natural disasters he has spent his life chasing die away to be replaced by the solid stability of parenthood.

This type of happy ending, in which the man promises his long-term and exclusive care, is the third major dimension of female desire, and one which, from an evolutionary point of view, makes perfect sense. An attraction to handsome men can make women more likely to produce genetically healthy children; an attraction to rich men can make them more likely to furnish those children with a good start; but an attraction to men who will stick around, be faithful, and dedicate themselves to protecting and nourishing their families over the long term is in many ways the most useful attraction pattern of all. Perhaps it's no coincidence that one of the best-selling photographic images of the 1980s showed a semi-nude male model, Adam Perry, cradling a tiny baby. Pictures of Adam alone sold steadily, but once he was shown devoting himself to a child, his career rocketed. Unfortunately, as in so many sexual battlefields, his image on paper didn't match his behaviour in real life. Perry was recently reported to have profited from the image in more than monetary terms: it had enabled him to seduce many of the three thousand women he claims to have slept with over the last ten years.

This evidence is, of course, anecdotal. But Bruce Ellis, now at the Vanderbilt University in Tennessee, has done a considerable amount of academic work on the parameters for male attractiveness, and claims to have found a preliminary link between the amount of time men spend 'investing' in their women and the frequency with which those women experience orgasm. And Peggy La Cerra, in a parallel study to the one in which women were shown to prefer men in high-status clothes to men in low-status clothes, has now shown that men who are photographed smiling at babies consistently receive higher attractiveness ratings from women than men who are photographed either ignoring babies or on their own. Female desire really did seem to be zeroing in on men who could deliver the guarantee of satisfaction: lasting, loving commitment to their partners and their children. The ideal of the New Man is not an invention of the sentimental late twentieth century; it's the rediscovery of a primal female fantasy.

Unfortunately, real-life Harlequin heroes and rich, handsome superdads are very thin on the ground, and for good reasons. Bearing in mind that inside every man is a polygynist waiting to get out, the call for extra-pair sex has rarely gone unanswered, especially by the rich and powerful. From the early despots, through today's pop stars, playboys and politicians to the chisel-jawed likes of Adam Perry, powerful, resource-laden and exceptionally handsome men have consistently had more sexual partners than the rest – simply because they can.

In the face of these odds, the woman's evolutionary ideal of a life of tender, loving care from a single perfect man would seem doomed. Doomed, that is, unless it had been backed up by some rather more practical fall-back strategies. For it now seems that evolution, the ultimate pragmatist, has actually taken women down a rather more complex path.

Inside the Volksgarten

Inside the Volksgarten, the atmosphere is dense and heavy. Cigarette smoke curls through the beams of the spotlights, which twist and spin around the room picking out dancers like acrobats in a blacked-out circus tent. In the middle of the floor, Sophie dips and thrusts to the visceral beat of the latest house and garage sounds. This is the twentieth-century techno mating-ground, one of the most popular night-clubs in Vienna. And tonight, it's business (and pleasure) as usual, except for one thing.

In a small basement underneath the main dance floor, researchers from the University of Vienna are examining the behaviour of the female clubbers. One by one, they are asked to come down and spit into a small, plastic vial, which is then sealed, logged, and taken back to the laboratory for examination. The researchers then ask them what sort of mood they are in, how many people arrived at the club with them, and whether or not they are in an established relationship. A video camera moves up and down their clothes as their answers are recorded. After about five minutes, they are free to leave. The experiment has been devised by Professor Karl Grammer, a groundbreaking urban ethologist who has made it his business to examine whether, and to what extent, evolutionary forces affect contemporary human behaviour. Today, he's exploring the relationship between female sexuality and the major hormones which lie behind it.

Ever since hormones were first discovered in the 1920s, scientists have suspected that they play a vital role in shaping our sex drive, exerting a powerful influence on the frequency with which we become aroused, the types of arousal we experience, and even the sorts of people who excite us. The male sex drive, as we have seen, is chiefly governed by a relatively stable level of testosterone, inclining its owner towards frequent sexual activity with a wide variety of women. The female sex drive, on the other hand, is influenced by a complex mixture of three very different hormones: oestrogen, testosterone, and progesterone.

Debates have raged for the last fifty years over exactly how these hormones exert their effect, and when. One camp argues that they have very little influence, especially in comparison with the massive social and cultural pressures traditionally foisted on women. Others suggest that hormone levels and balances vary so much from woman to woman that no meaningful generalisations can be made. Still a third group proposes that, because research into the relationship between hormones and desire is still relatively new, no hard and fast conclusions should yet be drawn. The real picture is far from clear, yet trends are emerging which allow us to provide initial, if somewhat tentative, sketches. So, for the purposes of simplicity, let us collect the evidence and sum up what we know of the ebb and flow of each hormone over a woman's monthly cycle, together with its basic psychological profile.

The first hormone we need to examine is oestrogen, which is produced throughout the month but which peaks just prior to ovulation. The sex therapist Theresa Crenshaw calls oestrogen the 'Marilyn Monroe' hormone; the come-here-and-touch-me, take-me-I'm-yours, kissing and squeezing hormone responsible for creating a woman's very femaleness; her rounded breasts and curvy hips, and her yearning for sexual contact.

The second major hormone is testosterone, which is produced in far smaller quantities by women than by men, but which rises to its highest level right around ovulation, where it appears to have much the same effect as for males. Testosterone is the prowler in the night, the sportsman running for touchdown, the businessman closing his deal; the active, aggressive urge to chase, fight and conquer. And this applies to the sexual arena too. Testosterone doesn't lie back and think of England. It gets up and gets into the game.

The final one of these three major hormones is progesterone, best known for its dampening effect. Progesterone is the wet blanket of the trio, encouraging women to stay at home and guard their privacy.

Those who are high in progesterone, which rises towards the end of the monthly cycle, as well as during pregnancy, typically display nurturing and defensive rather than active and aggressive behaviour.

When we consider this array of potent chemicals working in concert, ebbing and flowing in complementary patterns over the course of each monthly cycle, a new and far more sophisticated picture of female sexual desire begins to emerge.

Let's revisit Sophie, whom we met just now in the Viennese night-club. According to her report, Sophie is twenty-six and involved in a long-term relationship. On the night she visited the club, her boyfriend was at home, but while he felt tired and lethargic she had been restless. She resolved to go out on her own, slipped into a little black dress, and this is where she ended up. She had no particular plans to meet anyone, but she dressed for the occasion all the same. Soon, Sophie found herself being approached by a number of different men, and she was tempted to respond. By the time the researchers found her, she was in full swing – her head thrown back, her dress riding high, and a dangerous glint in her eyes.

The researchers who had been questioning Sophie were finding this an increasingly common pattern. Not just the preponderance of women in relationships who happened to arrive on their own, but also the way they behaved and the styles of clothing they wore. When they analysed Sophie's spittle sample, they were even more interested. It was very high in both oestrogen and testosterone. She was ovulating.

Putting together her style of dress, her hormonal state, and the circumstances under which she had arrived at the club, the researchers found the following pattern: Sophie, like a disproportionate number of other women at the club that night, was away from her boyfriend, maximally fertile, and dressed more skimpily than nearly all those who were not ovulating. The study doesn't record whether Sophie had sex with a different man that night, but it doesn't matter. Under the influence of her hormones, she was driven to behave in such a way that she might, and to do so just at the point when she was most likely to conceive. The question is, why?

Sperm wars

In April 1989, the British women's magazine *Company*, which is aimed at upwardly mobile professional women, launched a survey entitled 'The Orgasm: Your Chance to Redefine It'. Over the pages that followed, readers were invited to reveal some very specific information about their sexual experiences. The questionnaire wanted to know how often women had sex, with whom, at which times of the month, under what circumstances, what kind of contraception they used, and whether and when they climaxed. On the surface, it was a questionnaire like many others. But there was one notable difference. The questions in this one had not been compiled by a hurried editorial assistant, but by two of the country's most forward-thinking biologists.

Robin Baker and Mark Bellis were two maverick scientists feeling their way towards a radical new theory about female sexuality. Since the early 1980s, Baker had been working with biologist Geoffrey Parker on a phenomenon in the animal world known as sperm competition, in which the ejaculates from two different males were thought to combat each other inside the reproductive tracts of females in a sort of race to inseminate them. After changing direction for a while, when he took to studying spatial orientation and dizziness, Baker returned to the subject of sexuality and teamed up with his postgraduate student, Bellis, in a project that was to have an enormous impact – not just on the academic community, but on the whole institution of sex research.

Starting with some of the more ruthless facts of biology, like sperm competition, had given Baker and Bellis a new perspective on the controversy over female sexuality. They noted that in other primates testicle size (in relation to the whole body weight) varied according to how much control males had over 'their' females' mating habits. In polygynous species where a male dominated a harem of females (gorillas, for example), testicles were relatively small. In more egalitarian species, where both sexes were promiscuous, testicle size was far larger – most notably in our near-relatives the bonobo chimpanzees. Yet human testicle size fell somewhere in between – suggesting very strongly to Baker and Bellis that we evolved in conditions where men had to adapt to mild but consistent female philandering.

If males were responding to female tactics by evolving organs to match, and even by competing inside the reproductive tracts of females, did females themselves have any biological tools with which to influence the outcome? This was the central question, and from its very direct premise, Baker and Bellis were about to get closer than any researcher before them to solving the remaining great unknowns about female sexuality. Why was it so variable, what was the real function of the clitoris, and why should women have orgasms at all?

To get some depth as well as breadth into their results, Baker and Bellis recruited two groups of women. The first group – women who were involved in relationships – were asked to record in some detail the movements of sperm inside their reproductive tracts. How much was produced, how long did it stay there, and how much trickled out afterwards? Perhaps not surprisingly, this aspect of the sexual process had not been studied before. No one considered it an interesting or significant phenomenon, and even if they had, they might have wished to stay clear of it. But Baker and Bellis were acting on a hunch, and they thought that this apparently unaesthetic phenomenon might be a key to understanding human mating. They even gave it a name: 'flowback'.

Eleven couples were found, most of them undergraduates at the university and all in monogamous relationships. The couples were asked to carry on their sex lives as usual, but with two significant differences. First, each partner should record the timings of his or her orgasms, and second, the women should collect whatever fluids trickled from their vaginas after the sexual act, and place them in containers with chemical fixatives. This flowback was to be delivered to the researchers as soon as possible for analysis. The second group of subjects was much larger, and their task was considerably easier. All they had to do was answer the *Company* questionnaire. The results of the two studies were then analysed together and, amazingly, the following pattern emerged.

First, the amount of fluid which emerged from the vagina after sex wasn't always the same – and it didn't depend on the volume of the man's ejaculate. Rather, the amount of flowback varied with the timing of the female orgasm. If a woman climaxed any time from one minute before the man to three minutes afterwards, more sperm was retained in her vagina than if she climaxed much earlier than him, or much later, or not at all.

Second, although only about 20 per cent of the women's orgasms had occurred during vaginal intercourse (the remaining 80 per cent being achieved by masturbation, fantasy, or foreplay), the frequency of these copulatory orgasms was by far the highest when they were maximally fertile, around ovulation. Perhaps, suggested Baker and Bellis, the ancient Greeks had been on the right track, even if their ideas were flawed. Maybe a woman's orgasm during or around sexual intercourse really does play a role in conception. But what sort of role, and how?

Since Masters and Johnson had made their observations in the 1960s, and since Gorm Wagner at the University of Copenhagen had actually filmed the process of female orgasm in the vagina during the 1970s, researchers had noticed a unique physiological effect. They called it 'tenting'. As the muscles of the vagina and uterus contract, the rear wall of the vagina rhythmically shudders upwards, while the tip of the cervix dips down repeatedly. This creates a suction effect, so that whatever fluid may be pooled in the vagina – either sperm or the woman's own secretions – is drawn up through the entrance of the cervix. For sperm, this gives a real kick-start to the journey into the fallopian tubes to find and fertilise an egg. It also gets them out of the vagina, which while it might be a comfortable environment for a penis, is actually rather hostile to individual sperm. The pH balance of a healthy vagina is slightly acid, and mildly spermicidal. Once through the cervix, though, conditions are far more conducive to sperm survival. The process was a delicate one, but was given an unlovely name: 'upsuck'. Having established how much sperm the women were retaining, and under what circumstances, Baker and Bellis then had to identify exactly whose sperm it was. To accomplish this, they first had to do the maths: ascertain how often women were having sex when they were fertile, and with whom.

The survey results revealed that 47 per cent of respondents had 'double-mated', meaning that they had had sex with more than one man within a five-day period, at least once. This seemed to tally with other findings about women's choice of sexual partner. As early as 1948, Kinsey's team had found that 8 per cent of young wives had engaged in extramarital affairs, rising to 20 per cent by the age of thirty-five. As young women's sexual freedom increased over the decades, the figures rose. In 1980, a *Cosmopolitan* survey showed that of married women under thirty-four, half admitted they'd been unfaithful. This increased to 70 per cent for those women over thirty-five. Admittedly, readers of *Company* or *Cosmopolitan* might have been more sexually informed, more sexually active, and more willing to tell than the average woman – especially those self-selectors who'd choose to fill out a sex survey. But with figures like these, it was becoming increasingly difficult to argue that women were inherently less sexually active or variety-seeking than men.

But if these figures were already beginning to chip away at the cherished ideal of female monogamy, Baker and Bellis soon found another result which was even more revealing. Women were most likely to have sex with their regular partners in the first and last week of their menstrual cycles, and least likely to have sex with them in the middle of the cycle, when they were most likely to get pregnant. On the other hand, those women who had lovers were most likely to meet them on the days when they were most fertile. This is exactly what Karl Grammer's Viennese night-club experiment had shown. During those fertile days, when oestrogen and testosterone were highest, women would be most keen to seek and find sexual satisfaction, and most willing to do so outside of an established relationship.

And testosterone didn't just stimulate sexual intercourse. It spurred women to masturbate too. Far from the popular stereotype of frustrated, lonely women giving themselves what pleasure they could, studies consistently showed that the more sex women were getting, the more they masturbated. It wouldn't be surprising if the rush of sexual excitement from finding a lover might account for part of this. But could there be a more covert reason too? Baker and Bellis suggested that, bearing in mind the pH balance of vaginal fluid and the sucking effects of orgasm, episodes of masturbation would effectively put the drawbridge up for the next cargo of sperm, providing an acidic environment not just inside the vagina but right up past the cervix.

The chances of fertilisation didn't look good for the regular partner's sperm. But Baker and Bellis found the picture was even gloomier when they factored in the other crucial information. They now knew when women were having sex. They wanted to know how as well. It soon emerged that regular partners were at a double (or even triple) disadvantage. Even if a woman was having sex with both her partner and her lover during the days she was fertile, her orgasms were much more often synchronised with those of her lover than with those of her regular partner, with corresponding effects on the amount of sperm retained. Seventy per cent of fertile liaisons with lovers were of the high-retention type, compared with only 40 per cent of those with regular partners. The odds really were stacked in favour of the sneak. In fact, it turned out that a woman could have sex with her husband twice as often as with her lover, yet still shift the probability of paternity in favour of her lover.

Robin Baker, in particular, is not one for believing that human beings make decisions about anything, especially their sex lives, through pure logic. He's convinced that we're very largely under the sway of evolutionary drives we may not be even aware of, let alone able to balance up and compute. According to him, our bodies do a lot of the thinking for us, and we might have altogether too flattering a picture of our powerful brains. And this is where one of the most surprising findings of the *Company* study comes in. Given the incredible risks of being found out, you might think that women would be extra-careful about contraception if they were fooling around. Yet experience tells us this isn't always the case. Even lovers who've concocted the most elaborate strategies for getting out of the house and meeting in secret have 'slipped up' when it comes to contraception. They're obviously capable of assessing risk and acting intelligently. So why the lapse?

Baker and Bellis found that when women had 'double-mated' they were more likely than average to have used no contraception at all. Women who double-mated were much less likely to be on the pill. And they were much less likely to use contraception with the outsider than with their regular partner.

All the evidence pointed to a single conclusion. Women, just as much as men, were designed to get the very best genetic deal they could – and if that deal wasn't available within a relationship, they were all too prepared to get it elsewhere. As some sociobiologists wryly noted as they wrestled with the problem of female sexuality, the male urge for varied, extra-pair sex would never have survived if at least some women hadn't obliged them through the evolutionary process. And it couldn't all be to do with extracting resources. Women were also after something much more enduring – genes.

Whether or not they are consciously aware of what is going on in their bodies, women have been equipped with an armoury of tools for manipulating the paternity of their children: concealed ovulation; internal fertilisation; flowback; upsuck; masturbation; orgasm – all were ways of tipping the balance in favour of one man or another, without being too obvious about it. In this context, the roles of the clitoris and the female orgasm were far from mere coincidences of mammalian evolution. They gave women *power*. And those who understood even part of the process could have made more conscious choices. Tim Taylor, an archaeologist from the University of Bradford, has suggested that flowback may have been even more crucial in our evolutionary past, when regular strenuous exercise (and a notable lack of chairs) equipped our female ancestors with strong and controllable pubic muscles. Early women may have been able not just to let sperm drain out, but actively to expel it.

Cads and Dads

Yet a central question remains. Why risk it? If the processes of reproduction that couldn't be avoided – pregnancy, lactation and childcare – were so exhausting and risky in themselves, why multiply the dangers by choosing to be unfaithful? There was plenty of sperm around, and male jealousy was violent and widespread enough to be a real deterrent. But somehow it never seemed to stop extra-pair sex. Women were ready to balance the extreme risks of discovery against the advantages of a set of good genes. What could possibly explain this?

Men's desire for variety, and the imbalance in parental investment, could have left women in a no-win situation. Women need resources to survive and raise children. But men who have resources aren't necessarily those with the best genes. It's so hard, as women today lament, to find it all in one package. This problem has probably become more complicated over time, with more elaborate ways of earning a living that don't depend only on strength or cunning. But it seems to have been a dilemma for most of human history. Who will you choose? The steady, reliable provider? Or the penniless hunk who makes your heart skip a beat?

Of course, in our ancestral environment, men with resources were pretty likely to be the biggest, the strongest, and possibly the healthiest and most attractive too. This made life no easier for women. Guys with good genes would be even more unlikely than the average male to stick to one woman. It wasn't only men who would have to compete by any means possible to find themselves the best possible chance of reproductive success. Women would have to compete just as fiercely, just as cunningly, if rather less violently, for the best possible mate and the best share of the spoils. In polygynous communities, getting the best was even more complicated. Life in the harems might have been fun for the despots, but for the women it was a constant struggle for power, for resources, and even for survival. Women may well have preferred to find an averagely good resource provider to take care of their offspring, and reap the genetic benefit of sex with more dashing men when they could.

It's all oddly reminiscent of the male mixed strategy: find a partner, settle down to ensure at least some children live, and pursue alternative avenues when the costs aren't too high. Is it possible that there are similar psychological adaptations for weighing up the options in both sexes?

David Buss thinks there are. In his study on long- and short-term mating, which brought some of the more unedifying aspects of male choice to light, women also let slip some of their priorities. We've already seen how men divided women into 'good girls' and 'bad girls', and made their bets for long- or short-term mating accordingly. And we remember how far, for purposes of sex, men would drop their standards to levels which women were never willing to plumb. It all seemed to show that men were urgent and women were coy; men were keen and women were choosy. But closer examination shows that women were actually playing a mirror image of the same short-term game. They were dividing men up into 'dads' and 'cads', the male equivalents of 'madonnas' and 'whores'.

Buss explained many of his findings by saying that, while men short-term mated just for the sexual opportunities (hence their lower standards), the imbalance in parental investment just didn't make it worthwhile for women to pursue short-term mating as an end in itself. Women tended to do it for other reasons: 'Immediate extraction of resources, using short-term mating as an assessment device to evaluate long-term prospects, [and] securing protection from abuse by non-mated males . . .' That's what women were really after in a short-term partner. So indices of his readiness to spend and invest would be particularly important. Indeed, when asked about the qualities they'd find attractive in a short-term partner, women did respond very positively to lavish spending and very negatively to early stinginess.

Other findings, however, seemed to suggest that different reasons were at work – some of them in exact reverse to the general trend. While women were consistently choosier than men, even about short-term partners, like men they were pickier about long-term partners than occasional ones. This makes sense for both sexes, of course. It's a lot easier to accept someone for a few hours a week than for the rest of your life. Oddly enough, though, when it came to physical attractiveness, women drastically reversed their own pattern for demanding more of a long-term partner. For example, they placed much greater value on physical strength in a short-term than a long-term mate. They were also more exacting about physical attractiveness in short-term partners. As well as contradicting their own trends, women here also showed their difference from men, who as we recall were willing to drop their physical standards for casual flings. If you want to jump into bed with me without any investment or commitment, the women seemed to be saying, you really are going to have to be exceptionally attractive. We're back to the Diet Coke hunk.

Women, it seemed, were perfectly capable of balancing good genes against resources and commitment, and genes were sometimes the winner. Buss's initial emphasis on resource extraction also took a battering from other rather astonishing results. Women actually didn't appear to care too much whether short-term partners were poor, uneducated, or unambitious – although these were massive handicaps to potential long-term choices. Moreover, women rated qualities like 'has a promising career', 'likely to succeed in his profession', 'has a reliable future career' and 'likely to earn a lot of money' as less than half as important for short-term partners as they would be for long-term choices. Young men without resources might have more chances with women than they thought, as long as those women had already set up a flow of resources from somewhere else.

All this points to a radical new explanation of the female sex drive. For all those years during which researchers were seeking to categorise women, proverbially speaking, either as madonnas or whores, they were basing their ideas on a fundamental misconception: that the two categories were mutually exclusive, that no madonna could be a whore and no whore a madonna. Perhaps men thought that by tying female sexuality down to a neat binary formula, they would be better equipped to control it, even if their formula at times patently disregarded at least half the evidence. If women were all madonnas, why worry about providing them with pleasure? If they were all whores, at least measures could be taken to control their wayward inclinations. What's more, such measures could be justified. But if they were *both* – depending on their mood, the time of the month, the men presented to them, and any number of other factors – then what chance did a man have?

What chance indeed. Evolution has not designed men and women to live in calm, untroubled harmony, but to take whatever steps are necessary to load the dice in favour of optimum gene propagation for the individual. Men and women are fundamentally different when it comes to sex. Given the imbalance in the costs of reproduction, it's easy to see how we believed for so long that men were built for maximum polygyny, and women for secure monogamy. But we were wrong. Men and women are locked into an incremental evolutionary arms race, where their interests can seem irreconcilable. In a world of limited resources, limited energy and vital competition, there is inevitably some sort of 'battle of the sexes'. Yet the warring sides have more in common than they think. Both labour under biological handicaps: the mystery of paternity, the danger of pregnancy. Both have biological drives and tools to offset these handicaps and further their genes: men's gigantic sperm capacity and desire for variety, women's orgasms and maternal care. Both have sophisticated psychological mechanisms for weighing up the potential of lasting and temporary partners.

And however uncomfortable we may be in coming to terms with it, however incomprehensible the opposite sex may seem at times, both men and women are adapted for one basic pattern: long-term relationships to raise secure offspring, peppered with sex on the side.

PART TWO

SHAPING FORCES

*Social controls on sexual behaviour. Why they arose and
how they have shaped the sexuality of the West.*

3

The Road to Marriage

In 1937, Helena Valero was abducted. The daughter of a Spanish frontiers-man who had ventured into the spectacular Brazilian rainforests between the Rio Grande and Upper Rio Orinoco, Helena was a resourceful and resilient child, but nothing had prepared her for the day of the attack. Her small family was paddling their canoe towards a deserted house in which they had been planning to set up home, when they saw smoke rising from a nearby clearing. They headed for the bank and Helena's father stepped ashore to investigate. Two minutes later, he was sprinting back, stricken with panic and with an arrow through his arm. 'There are Indians,' he cried. 'Indians! Drop the baggage! Get paddling!'

The family jumped into the canoe and raced off downstream, but the Indians gave chase, unleashing wave after wave of arrows. One scraped past Helena's stomach and embedded itself in her thigh. For a moment the Valeros thought they were getting away, but a formation of rocks loomed in front of them. Along it stood a long line of warriors, their bows and spears at the ready. Now desperate, the family abandoned ship and leapt into the rapids. They scrambled ashore and tried to run for cover, but Helena's two young brothers couldn't carry themselves fast enough and Helena, deeply wounded by the arrow, could hardly walk. Picking up the boys, Helena's parents ran into the forest, shouting to their daughter that they would be back.

The next thing Helena knew, it was night-time and she was lying by a fire in the heart of the Indian village. It was the beginning of a lengthy odyssey in which she was to learn the ways of one of the last 'undiscovered' tribes on Earth.

The Yanomamo, as they were called, lived in groups of about fifty people, centred around fortified villages deep in the jungle. They ate spiders, toads, snakes and, for ceremonial purposes, the ashes of their dead relatives. The women wore bones through their noses, the men sported penis guards, and both sexes decorated their bodies with a red paste called *urucu*.

Helena watched with wonder the customs of her adoptive people, which included ritual slapping matches, shamanic dancing, and the use of trance-inducing drugs. When she reached puberty, Helena too was caught up in the rituals. Suddenly she was taken by two women and forced inside a bamboo cage, where she was left with very little food or drink for several weeks. At the end of this period, she was washed, dressed, painted and paraded through the village to signal her entry into womanhood. She was now, as the Yanomamo put it, a woman 'of consequence', and men began to take an interest in her. Her name spread beyond the confines of the village, and soon a potential husband with a party of warriors came to spirit her away.

Yanomamo marriages seemed to have little in common with the wooing and seductions of the West. They were often the result of violent raids, when warriors descended on neighbouring villages, killed or disabled the men, dashed out the brains of the children, and carried away the screaming women. Although the man who had come to claim Helena was less warlike, he was no gentler. Helena described her experience:

> I was lying in the hammock; I saw lots of men, all painted. The first one came up with his arrows in his hand and stood still looking. I turned my face towards the shapuno roof; I wanted to escape through the leaves of the roof. The man who stood in front of all the others dropped his arrows and took me by the arm. I was still turning my head towards the roof. The man said, 'I have come to take her.'

At this point, the old women of Helena's village were reluctant to lose her. A tug-of-war ensued over her body, with the warriors trying to drag her away by the legs and the old women clinging on to her by the neck. Eventually, Helena passed out and was left for dead. She'd escaped capture, and was eventually married to the village headman, Fusiwe, who already had four other wives.

Unfortunately, as Helena would find out, relations between co-wives were often strained. She once witnessed a new wife wandering non-chalantly back from a liaison in the woods with her husband, only to be violently attacked by his senior wife, waving a stick. These sorts of altercations were frequent and often bloody. Sometimes the husband stood by and watched, sometimes he took part, giving one or both wives a beating.

Life with Fusiwe was hard. Helena's co-wives were jealous, and Fusiwe himself was brutal, falling into a furious rage if any of them went to sit by his brother's fire, and beating them regularly about the head. Helena bore Fusiwe two sons before he fell prey to a raiding party; she found her way to a new group and was allocated to the cruel and malevolent Akawe, who continually threatened to kill her. Many years had now passed since she had arrived, he said. She was too old to be attractive any more and her age prevented him from enjoying the company of younger women. Helena endured his insults and beatings for what were to be her final years in the jungle. Then, at a time when she felt herself most in danger, a Venezuelan trading ship came by and she managed to get herself aboard. Four days later, she arrived in Rio. The papers heard about her story and wrote about this white woman's life with the savages in terms resembling those used by today's most lurid tabloids. But why the fascination?

Helena had survived an extraordinary adventure, but her tale was more complex, more powerful, and more telling than the usual hackneyed yarns of women in peril. She had not only lived with these people, learning about their ways from the outside. She had lived as they did, observing their rituals and marrying in their tradition. But what was the real meaning of her experience? Was it just a nightmarish traveller's tale of a savage people, as different from the 'civilised' world as night is from day? Was the constant violence of Yanomamo society a strange aberration, created by the harsh conditions of jungle living? Or was the really shocking thing about Helena's story its very familiarity? Could it be that her experience was really just an extreme example of a disturbingly familiar global pattern – the archetype of all marital arrangements?

Delighting in difference

The idea that human sexual relations follow essentially the same pattern all over the world strikes most anthropologists as absurd. From the time

when human beings first set out across the oceans to conquer new peoples
and explore new lands, they have always delighted in telling tales of their
differences, and never more so than in the sexual sphere. In the ancient
world, the Romans recorded with wide-eyed fascination the Egyptian
habit of royal incest. In the Middle Ages, the Spanish conquistadors
filled their diaries with reports of sodomy and transvestism among the
Incas; and in Victorian times, when missionaries set out to spread God's
word among the 'savage' peoples of Africa, Asia and Oceania, breathless
reports of gang rape, institutionalised paedophilia, the ritual defloration of
virgins, sexual slavery, and widow immolation soon followed.

The accent on difference, although given a new spin of 'non-judge-
mental' reporting, has continued in more recent times. The discipline of
anthropology thrives on discovering, explaining and often promoting the
peculiarities of different tribes and cultures. Fieldworkers have a magnetic
attraction to societies with norms as far removed as possible from the
contemporary West. Writing accounts of people with radically different
sexual or marital practices is a sure-fire ticket to success, bound to spread
the fame and reputation of the scholar.

Thus, we have been told, there is a society in the Pacific which knows
nothing of the pains and pleasures of romantic love; another, on the great
plains of North America, where sexual jealousy is effectively banished;
and a third, in West Africa, where women are richer and scarcer than
men, calling the sexual shots and leisurely choosing the sexual services
of respectful and obedient males. In a world plagued by media reports
of marital violence, romantic heartache and sexual disappointment, such
cultures seem to offer an elusive glimpse of a better, happier world. If
sexual life can be so radically re-arranged, we think, no sexual problem
can be insoluble.

But the more these cultures are revisited and re-examined, the less
such differences stand up to scrutiny. In some cases, customs have been
misinterpreted by investigators, who looked in the wrong places and
asked the wrong questions; in others, anthropologists were so anxious
to make a name for themselves that occasional events were trumpeted
as major cultural institutions, and exceptions blithely interpreted as the
rule. Then, too, missionaries eager to promote the precepts of their own
faith were over-zealous in uncovering (or inventing) behaviour which they
could decry as ungodly and unjust, the proven justification for instant
conversion.

The 'natives' so described were not always innocent bystanders in this process. In one famous example, the Trobriand Islanders misled world-famous anthropologist Bronislaw Malinowski into believing that they had no idea that sex led to conception, leaving him to publish on the subject before revealing that they knew perfectly well where babies came from. In another example, the claim that the Mangaian Islanders engaged in epic bouts of sex but had no concept of romantic love turned out to be a hoax: a shattering anthropological revelation had been drawn from nothing more than the drunken bragging of a group of village boys.

In the first part of this book I hope I have shown that there is something approaching a universal sexual nature. In this part, I hope to suggest that there is a fundamental sexual *culture*, formed over the last 30,000 years, which reflects and builds on human nature, moulding itself to suit the demands of different landscapes, different population distribution and the technologies of different peoples – but constant in shape and texture underneath. It is this human sexual culture which has shaped the history of the world's great civilisations, allowing some to flourish and others to wither, and which continues to shape ourselves and our sexuality today.

An uncanny feeling

Consider the following true story. Terri and Kim met in June 1985, when they were in their late twenties. It was a beautiful summer's day. Hazy sunshine, the air laced with the peculiarly British smell of budding roses and freshly mown lawns. Terri was wandering around the house, setting things straight and getting ready for her sister, who was due to arrive for lunch. A car drew up outside. Looking through the sitting-room window, Terri could see that her sister had arrived, and that she was accompanied by two men. One was her sister's boyfriend; the other, to Terri's astonishment, was their long-lost brother, Kim, separated from her family at birth and brought up by adoptive parents.

As soon as she clapped eyes on Kim, Terri was entranced. 'There was a surge of electricity,' she remembers, 'and I knew instantly that I loved him, beyond any sort of love that I'd ever imagined.' Kim felt the same way: 'When I met Terri the feeling was so powerful and emotional,' he reports. 'It was as if there was an invisible, unconscious sort of bonding between us, even before we'd spoken.'

Lunch passed without incident. Terri went back to her normal life, and Kim to his. But two weeks later, they met again. In late June, Terri was invited to a barbecue in Kim's home town, Southend. She rang and asked if she could spend a couple of nights with him. He was delighted. Terri arrived on the Friday evening and they had dinner together. The attraction was still there, now stronger than ever. 'We just stared at each other,' remembers Kim, 'and I felt as if I'd known her all my life. It was an uncanny feeling.'

After dinner, Kim showed Terri to her room, and they sat on the bed to talk. Slowly, they moved closer to each other, and shortly after midnight they shared their first kiss. It was a magical experience. Unable to resist each other any longer, they undressed and climbed into bed.

On one level, it was a dream come true. Here were two ordinary people who had found an extraordinary love. But on another plane, the story of Terri and Kim was a nightmare which had only just begun. First, Terri's sister turned up at her house and started shouting at her. 'You're sick. How could you?' She told them that she would never speak to them again unless they broke up. They didn't.

A few months later, Terri became pregnant. She and Kim were over-joyed, but few others saw cause for celebration. There were whispers that the baby would be retarded, or deformed, or both. Then, as soon as their child, a beautiful baby girl called Lisa, was born, Terri and Kim began to feel they were being watched. A week later, there came a knock at the door. It was the police. The couple were taken away to the station and questioned. They were shut in a cell for several hours, then released with a warning. What they had done was disgusting, dangerous and illegal. Terri should be sterilised and the couple would be well advised to live apart. And if not? If not, their baby would be taken away from them and they could be imprisoned for up to seven years.

Terri felt she had no choice. Hoping that the authorities would leave them alone, she booked herself into hospital and had the operation. But the police came back again. Terri and Kim were re-arrested and taken to court, where they both received a suspended sentence and were told never to live as man and wife again.

For the last ten years, Terri and Kim have endured a precarious existence, living in the same house, looking after Lisa, but each with a separate bedroom and both under continuous surveillance. Their story reads like an episode from George Orwell's 1984, in which love and personal affection are banned and sexual reproduction is controlled by the state rather than the vagaries of individual desire. But it's not. It's a perfectly ordinary boy-meets-girl story, set very much in the real world. As it happens, it's taking place now, in Essex, but it could have happened at any time, in any place, in any civilisation throughout history, and people's reactions would have been the same, because Terri and Kim have broken one of the oldest and most profoundly felt of all human sexual regulations.

Incest, the act of having sex with someone to whom you're related, has been legislated against in almost every culture on Earth from the time when written records began. It is one of the earliest and perhaps the most pervasive of all human taboos, and has attracted a wide variety of sanctions, ranging from execution (ancient Babylon), through embracing a red-hot statue (ancient India) to roasting in nine different hells (ancient China).

Yet despite the universality of the taboo, some cultures have imposed much more stringent sanctions than others. The ancient Egyptians, for instance, allowed incestuous marriage among the ruling classes as the only practical way to keep the precious lands along the Nile from being dispersed among ever-enlarging, ever-outbreeding families. The Hebrews, at the opposite end of the spectrum, legislated against all forms of incest with an enthusiasm which bordered on the fanatical, partly in an attempt to distinguish themselves from the Egyptians, under whose hated rule they had lived for so long. Starting with the prohibitions handed down to Moses on Mount Sinai, which specified, 'You shall not uncover the nakedness of your sister . . . of your son's daughter or your daughter's daughter,' the early rabbis extended the circle of forbidden relationships into a spiralling network of ever more distantly related kin. By the time they had finished, they had gone well beyond the inner core of parents, children, grandchildren, uncles, aunts and first cousins whom most cultures tried to keep apart, and had even included a ban on sex with one's 'maternal grandmother's paternal brother's wife'.

But why the universal consternation over incest? Why ban it at all? Sex is a dangerous, unpredictable business in which one risks humiliation, rejection, and sometimes aggression as well. Why not confine it to those whom one knows and trusts, like family? It's true that some cultures do engage in certain forms of sexual contact between relatives: Yanomamo fathers could tickle and suck on the vulvas of their infant daughters without causing even a ripple of scandal. Among the Sirionó of South America, mothers traditionally calmed their infant sons by masturbating them or sucking on their penis.

On a larger scale, however, there are three very good reasons why cultures the world over have generally sought to deter or eliminate incestuous relationships in all but the most transient or tactical of circumstances. The first reason is that the family dynamic is complex and delicate enough without it being obliged to incorporate an altogether different form of relationship. The balance of power between parents and children makes inter-generational incest an obvious candidate for an abuse or an upset of power; the favouritisms, passions and jealousies induced by sex rarely mesh well with existing patterns of familial love and care.

Secondly, incest may have a harmful effect on the health and stability of peoples who practise it if they do so too often for too long. The entire rationale of sex, we must remember, is to keep shuffling new genes together so that predators and parasites will never have a uniform style of organism on which to prey. If, through repeated incestuous unions over many generations, a culture passes on a decreasingly diverse set of genes, current diseases will spread and new ones will find it easy to take hold. Indeed, in those very few micro-cultures where inbreeding has been the norm, either through choice or circumstance, the health of the population does appear to have suffered. On the tiny island of Tristan da Cunha in the South Atlantic, for example, where no new blood was imported to mate with the twenty-three original settlers nor any of their descendants for the six generations between 1827 and 1961, a notable decline in overall health was registered. Of the 267 people who populated the island in 1961, 4 had a hereditary blindness-producing disease, 6 more were carrying it, and a further 8 were potential carriers. Furthermore, researchers noted that the most inbred members of the population were generally less intelligent than the least inbred.

These are the sorts of fears that Terri and Kim's family were expressing when they suggested that their baby would be born deformed, yet Terri and Kim's own story is, paradoxically, good evidence for the third explanation for human incest taboos. Our ancient ancestors are unlikely to have been consciously aware of the genetic disadvantages of incest; but they didn't need to be, for they were fitted, as we are today, with a sophisticated evolutionary adaptation which programmes us from birth to avoid it.

One of the most striking things about the purist kibbutz system, which operated in parts of Israel between the 1940s and 1990s, was the way in which children were reared. Instead of being brought up by their biological parents, they were deposited in large communal nurseries where they were encouraged to bond intensely, to experiment sexually (if they wished) and, eventually, to create the next generation of kibbutz kids. It was a brave idea and a novel one, but the most remarkable thing about it was that, despite the intense bonding which went on and the lifetime friendships which were forged, not a single individual ever mated with someone who had grown up on the same kibbutz. When asked why, they replied that they simply weren't attracted to them. It seemed that the intense and repeated contact which each had with the other early in life actually extinguished rather than inflamed desire.

In almost all communities, of course, the children most likely to be brought up in close proximity with each other have been siblings, so an adaptation which discouraged individuals from mating with those with whom they had been raised would effectively be an adaptation for avoiding incest. When anthropologists have asked members of tribal societies whether they could feel attraction for their brothers or sisters, the most common response has not been the sort of fury which might indicate repressed desire, but rather laughter or bemusement. 'Of course I can, she's a woman' is the most typical form of response. 'But I just don't think of her that way. I mean, she's my sister. Who'd want to sleep with their sister?' Seen in this light, the story of Terri and Kim is the exception which proves the rule. The fact that they fell in love may only have been possible because they were brought up separately.

Aside from the social confusion created by incest, and the natural revulsion which people appear to feel towards it, there is yet another reason why cultures the world over have sought to eradicate incest, and it's perhaps the most significant reason of all. Incest lessens what we might term outcest. And outcest – the practice of mating with strangers – may have been the most vital factor in determining which early tribes would grow and flourish, and which would wither and perish.

Outcest demanded that people acquire sexual partners from a group different from their own. In the early history of humanity, there were two main ways of achieving this. One, as we have seen, was to steal partners from one's neighbours by force. This is the method still employed by the Yanomamo, and while it ensures that incestuous unions are avoided, it does little for the overall peace and prosperity of the culture. Indeed, on one level, the whole of Yanomamo society can be seen as a series of bloody internecine battles between one group and another in which women are continually herded back and forth, while their menfolk are whittled away by murder in the process.

Other, perhaps cannier, groups must have recognised that outcest could be practised in a more peaceful and profitable manner. By sending sexual emissaries to act as long-term partners for the members of a neighbouring group, they could forge friendly alliances with that group, sharing tips on which predators to avoid, the whereabouts of good game or grazing, and the likely hostility or friendliness of other nearby tribes. When circumstances demanded, it also gave them ready allies alongside whom they could fight or with whom they could merge. And in the early days of humanity, where competition for food and territory was intense, this capacity for merger may have been vital in determining which groups would prosper.

But if alliances between tribes were to be made by the sending of sexual emissaries, who would those emissaries be, and how would the system work?

The origins of marriage

In 1908, on the banks of the Danube some thirty miles upstream of Vienna, a railway worker dug up a curious small object from the sidings. About the size of his hand, it resembled the figure of a short, fat woman with a pudding-bowl haircut, large pendulous breasts and uncommonly heavy hips and thighs. Assuming that it was a freak of nature, a pebble which simply happened to resemble a woman, he was about to throw it away, but then decided to take the precaution of showing it to an archaeologist who was working on a site nearby.

The archaeologist took the 'pebble' back to Vienna, where, after consultation with his colleagues, he confirmed that it was the earliest and finest example of a number of little statues which had been emerging from the soil of Europe for some three decades. The first was found in a location known as the Pope's Grotto, near Bayonne in the south of France, and the second at the nearby Grimaldi Grottoes. With gentle irony, since they were unimpressed by the pulchritude of these figures, the French gave them the name of Venus, the Roman goddess of love. Thus the Austrian statue was given the evocative name of 'The Venus of Willendorf', after the town near where she had been uncovered.

Since 1908, nearly two hundred further Venus figurines have come to light, in finds ranging from the steppes of Russia in the east to the Spanish Pyrenees in the west. The figures are startling not just for the range of their distribution, but also for the consistency of their design. They have all been carefully carved, some out of limestone and others out of bone or greenstone; while some depict hair and clothes and others not, they nearly all share the same shape, with massively enhanced breasts, over-emphasised hips, and a keen concentration on the genital area. The pubic mound is clearly visible on all the figurines, and on some even the labia have been featured in glorious though exaggerated detail. Yet despite the attention their creators paid to the genital area, almost none of the Venuses have faces. Their heads are smooth and blank. Opinions vary widely as to who made them, and why.

The first suggestion is that they represent a sort of powerful matriarchal goddess, reflecting an age in which Woman reigned supreme as 'Giver-of-Life, Wielder of Death, and as Regeneratrix'. But none of the figures appears to be directly creating life, wielding death, or making regeneration possible. If anything, they seem passive and static, as well as faceless. And as we saw in the last chapter, archaeology gives little other evidence to support the idea that there was ever an age of matriarchal rule.

A second suggestion is that the figurines were Stone Age centrefolds, used by men to gaze at while masturbating. Since the discovery of a number of phallic objects which have been interpreted by archaeologists as dildoes (some of them double-ended), this explanation, though it remains fanciful, may not be as unlikely as it sounds. If female masturbatory aids have existed for 30,000 years, why not male ones as well?

The third, and perhaps the most compelling, suggestion, is that the Venus figurines were gifts, carved by the world's earliest husbands while awaiting the arrival of their wives. The women, who came from far-off tribes with their families and friends, would be joined to the men in a ceremony which would most probably have included singing, dancing, and the giving of gifts – including, perhaps, the figurines, which were a symbol of the men's skill and a presage of the hope of fertility. The figures were taken home by the parents, who cherished them as a reminder of their daughters, and who were better able to envisage their faces on the smooth, blank surface than the husbands who had never previously met them. This interpretation is no more firmly grounded in fact than the first two, but the idea that formalised outcest was taking place by 30,000 BC, and that it was women who acted as sexual emissaries, seems to make sense from a variety of perspectives.

While often being the most regular spoil of war, women have also tended to be the best symbols, and often the best catalysts, for peace. Also, if your chief aim was to enlist muscle power to aid in hunting or abet in pillaging, it was the muscle whom one had to please. It's not hard to imagine that young, nubile women would have been better equipped to create a favourable impression on the males of a neighbouring group than hairy, combative men. It's worth noting here that the Venus figurines are the only human-shaped sculptures in durable materials from the period. Men were painted on the cave faces and might have been depicted in other, more perishable media. But durable sculptures were always of women – and to many, this has the clear implication that while women, and images of women, could be traded and given, men simply could not.

The final supporting argument is that it would make less sense to break up established hunting groups, which relied on each other's skills and specialisations and which were chiefly comprised of men, than it would to separate gathering groups, who relied more on their own skills, and who were chiefly made up of women.

There is a certain amount of corroboration for this schema from the archaeological record, too. In the coastal settlement of Téviec, in north-west France, studies of human bones show that the men had been raised primarily on a local marine diet, and most of the women on an inland diet. The women had not grown up on seafood; they had arrived, or been brought, from further inland. Moreover, from the evidence of burial sites all over Europe from this period, we know that humans were already carrying out death ceremonies, often involving symbolic use of space and motifs. And wherever death ceremonies exist, we might reasonably expect the existence of other ceremonial rites of passage.

All these factors suggest that by about 30,000 years ago, some type of formalised intertribal marriage was already in existence, and that it was the women who were the incoming party. But while the idea and the practice of marriage may have developed to cement alliances between rival and potentially hostile groups, the arrival of nubile women from neighbouring tribes was also destined to create as many problems as it solved. Although

BASIC INSTINCTS

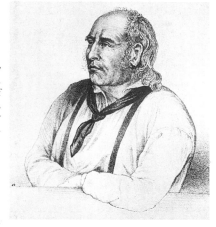

John Adams, the last surviving *Bounty* mutineer on the island of Pitcairn. Of the fourteen others, one died of natural causes, one committed suicide, and twelve were murdered in their struggle for the few available women.

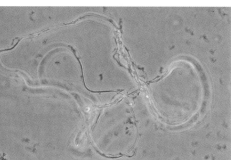

A light micrograph of DNA (deoxyribonucleic acid). It was strands like these, grouped together and hidden within a protective membrane of fats, which led to the evolution of all life-forms.

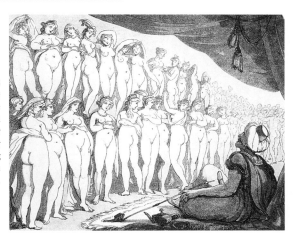

The Harem by Thomas Rowlandson. Wherever there have been resources to acquire and land to dominate, men have fought fiercely for supremacy, then directed their energies towards accumulating and enjoying the maximum number of women.

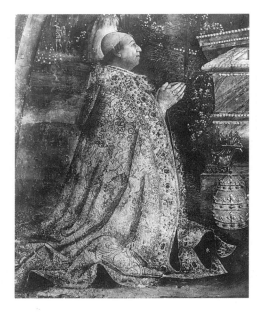

The pontiff as holy man:
Pope Alexander VI, better known
by his birth-name Rodrigo Borgia,
from the fresco by Pinturicchio in
the Borgia apartments of the Vatican.

The pontiff as beast: Borgia took
twenty-five prostitutes into his quarters
most nights, and arranged the infamous
'Joust of Whores', in which naked
women were obliged to race on all fours
down paths illuminated by candles, while
Borgia and his friends attempted to
mount whichever took their fancy.

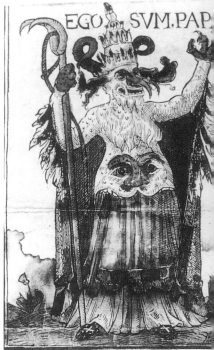

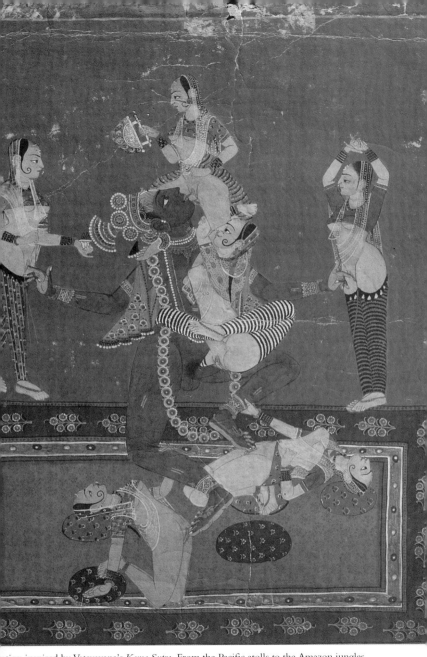

...ation inspired by Vatsyayana's *Kama Sutra*. From the Pacific atolls to the Amazon jungles, ...the wastelands of Waco to the royal palaces of Brunei, men have seen women as the currency, ...centive, and the reward of power.

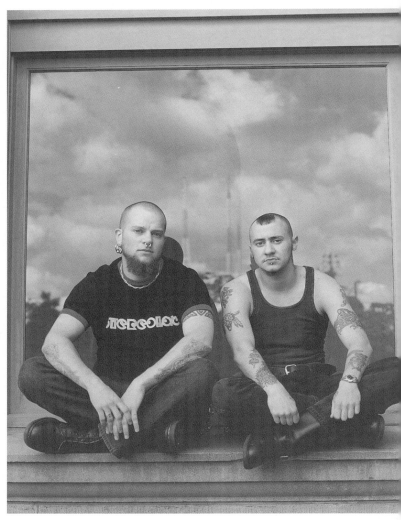

Matt and Eric, F-to-Ms from Seattle, Washington.

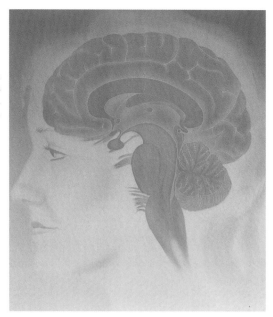

A cross-section of the human brain showing Paul MacLean's 'triune' hierarchy: brain stem, limbic system and cortex.

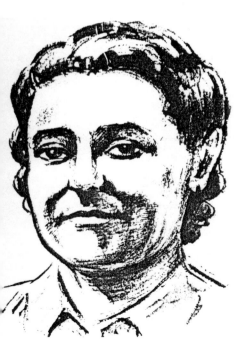

A sketch of Juliane Lipka, one of the murderesses of Nagyrev. Over one hundred men were killed in the village between 1914 and 1929 after their spouses had experienced real sexual freedom for the first time.

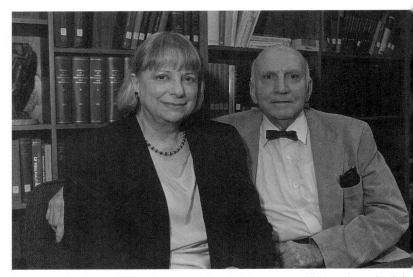

Husband-and-wife team William Masters and Virginia Johnson, who collaborated on a detailed examination of female sexuality whose results were published in their book *Human Sexual Response*.

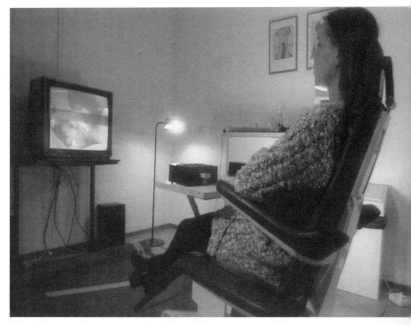

The University of Amsterdam's Sex Chair, which uses an array of instruments to measure the sex responses – both conscious and unconscious – of whoever sits in it.

The guarantee of satisfaction: Rita Clay Estrada's *The Stormchaser*, one of a series of highly successful romantic novels in which the hero always promises his long-term and exclusive care – a principal factor in female desire.

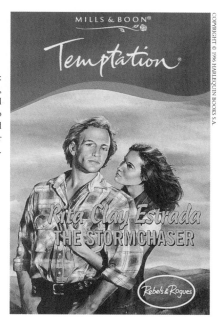

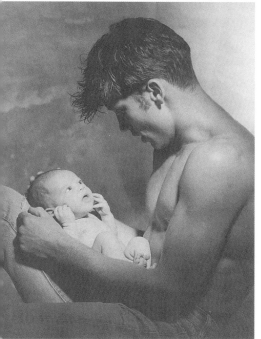

One of the best-selling images of the 1980s. Pictures of model Adam Perry on his own sold steadily, but once he got hold of the baby, sales rocketed.

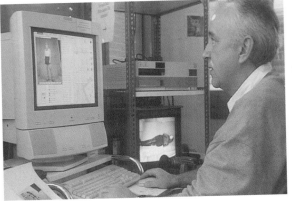

A female club-goer in Vienna being examined by Professor Karl Grammer. In a series of experiments Grammer found that women were most likely to be unfaithful on the very nights when they were most likely to conceive.

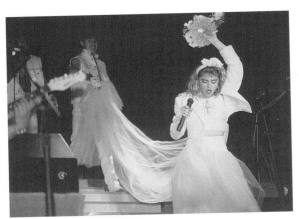

'Madonna' …

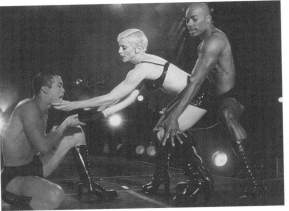

… or 'whore'? Actually, depending on their mood, the time of the month, the men presented to them, and any number of other factors, most women could be both.

it may have had a pacifying effect between tribes, it would have been potentially explosive within a tribe.

We've already seen how men are programmed to desire sex with the largest number of the most fertile women. They struggle and fight for sexual access, using either muscle power, brain power, or both. What we haven't yet seen is how men react when it's their own women to whom access is being sought. And this, in the early days of marriage, is exactly what was bound to happen. To her new husband, a woman was property. But to every other man she was potential prey.

The red threesome

High up in the Pavlov Hills of the northern Czech Republic lies the ancient settlement of Dolní Věstonice. It dates from around 20,000 years ago, at the height of the last Ice Age, when mammoths, bison and wild horses roamed the steppes of Eastern Europe. The inhabitants of Dolní Věstonice slept in hide tents, burned coal in their fireplaces, and dressed in skins and fur. We have no formal proof of the extent to which they had developed a distinct culture through which they administered their sexual and social organisations, their laws, customs, or religious beliefs; but we have some tantalising clues.

On the edge of the settlement is a shallow grave which contains the bodies of three young adults: a probable female flanked by two definite males. All had been cut off in their prime and buried together with what appears to be considerable ceremony. The man to the left has been carefully laid on his back, his head facing towards the central woman and his hands extending to touch her genitals. The woman, also on her back, is facing away from him towards the man on her right. This man, buried on his front, has his arm over the central woman's hand, but his head turned sharply away.

What had happened here? None of the bodies reveals any sign of disease or disfigurement which might hint at the cause of death. In any case, natural deaths in this area almost never resulted in burial. This was a special case. Looking more closely at the bodies yields some riveting clues. One can just discern traces of powder in the general region of the woman's genitals, and sprinkled over the heads of all three. The powder is red ochre. Furthermore, the coccyx of the man on the left, the one with his hands stretching over the woman's genitals, has been pierced with a sharp instrument, probably a spear.

There are several interpretations for this extraordinary burial. One is that the corpses were the victims of a human sacrifice; another is that they had committed a crime against the group. Bohuslav Klima, who excavated the site, believes that the burial may have followed a birth gone wrong, in which the two men are midwives and the woman an unfortunate mother. But there is little to suggest that men may ever have been more proficient at midwifery than women, and anyway, why the spear wound? A final interpretation, and one which appears to fit with all the evidence as well as being psychologically the most credible, is that this could be the first formal record of humanity's violent sanctions against adultery.

Following this framework, it is possible to see the woman in the centre as an errant wife, whose husband, to her right, has his arm stretched over her hand as a signal of proprietariness, but whose head is turned away in disgust. The man to the left is the sexual intruder, his hands extending towards her genitals to indicate the nature of their relationship, and his head turned towards her with desire. But who was killed by whom, and when? It is possible that the husband killed the wife's lover with the spear, and that the husband and wife were then both put to death by the rest of the tribe, with red ochre smeared over them to indicate that fertility was the issue at stake. Alternatively, the lover may have killed the husband, with the wife then being punished harshly by an outraged clan. Or the indiscretion may have been discovered by another member of the tribe, bringing a sentence of death to all three simultaneously.

Admittedly, this interpretation is like finding a hundred pieces from a thousand-piece jigsaw – we are left to guess at the other nine hundred pieces which might make a picture of prehistoric society. The very nature of sexual behaviour means that archaeology has few concrete things to tell us about prehistoric sexual *mores*. Nonetheless, the theme of adulterous intrusion by men, and the violent reprisals which ensued, echoes down the centuries to us today.

The green-eyed monster

The three classic sex manuals of world culture, Ovid's *Ars Amatoria*, Vatsyayana's *Kama Sutra*, and Sheikh Nefzawi's *Perfumed Garden*, all give copious advice on how to seduce other men's wives. Ovid, who was writing for an urbane Roman audience during the first century BC, recommends meeting her at the games, playing footsie under the table, and befriending her maid. Vatsyayana, whose *Kama Sutra* was composed two hundred years later, recommends suggesting picnics, sending presents, and making conspicuous show of one's love for her children. And Sheikh Nefzawi, writing for the Grand Vizier of Tunis in the sixteenth century, favours cutting a hole in the door of her house through which she can be penetrated.

But, as each of these authors knew, seducing other men's wives was a dangerous business. For since the time when marriage first came to exist, we have had to experience, and contend with, the jealous rage of the threatened husband.

For many years, in sociological literature at least, jealousy was held to be a 'secondary' emotion, somehow less fundamental and less important than the so-called 'primary' emotions of fear, anger, and disgust. Many even believed that it was the sign of an abnormal or unhealthy psychological constitution, and were fond of citing happier, more stable peoples like the Diere of south-east Australia, the Hidatsa of North America, and the Marquesa Islanders of the Pacific, where it was said not to exist.

Yet since the arrival on the academic scene of Martin Daly and Margo Wilson, a rather different picture has emerged. Daly and Wilson are a husband-and-wife team based at McMaster University in Canada, whose work has inspired a whole new generation of psychologists. Although they have delved into many of the seamier sides of human relations, from the abuse of stepchildren to the epidemiology of murder, they are primarily celebrated for their work on the evolution and effects of sexual jealousy.

Daly and Wilson hold that jealousy, far from being pathological and exceptional, is as fundamental to the human condition as eating, sleeping, and sexual desire. Although it may have unpleasant consequences, it is a vital part of our evolutionary make-up, for it is designed to prevent us being cheated or betrayed by the people in whom we need to place our greatest trust: the long-term sexual partners with whom we create and rear our children.

We know that, despite their good intentions, both men and women are designed to take advantage of each other; to pair up and then look for strategic mating opportunities on the side. We also know that while most people are all too ready to excuse their own cheating, they're much less tolerant of their partner's. While we may deplore the hypocrisy inherent in this situation, we can surely understand it.

From the man's point of view, his wife's sexual errantry may result in her returning to the marital bed having been impregnated with the sperm of another man. While this may be fine by her, it's disastrous for him. Genetically speaking, he could endure no more cruel fate nor suffer more fruitless a waste of time than to expend his energy and resources on bringing up another man's child in the mistaken belief that it was his own. He would have wasted the time, energy and resources that had gone into acquiring and maintaining her. He would have wasted whatever he had invested in her child. And he would have been unable to use her as a vehicle for passing on his own genes during the whole period of her pregnancy. Bearing in mind these heavy costs, evolution was likely to favour men who displayed a tendency to be vigilant over their partner's sexual activity and who were primed to react swiftly and decisively to any signs of straying. In other words, men who were jealous. And while on a day-to-day basis these tendencies might only surface on a minor level, they would blow up to epic proportions in response to real and concrete signs of infidelity or abandonment.

In such circumstances, a man's first reaction may well be targeted at the rival for his partner's affections. Indeed, research carried out by Daly and Wilson suggests that at least 20 per cent of all male/male homicides may have sexual jealousy as their root cause, even where, on the surface, the motive may seem to be something entirely different. But, as we know to our peril, men attack their wives too, sometimes with murderous results. In one study of women at a shelter for battered wives, nearly 50 per cent were targets of their husband's jealousy.

From a woman's point of view, her husband's errantry is just as serious. Although she always knows that the children she bears are hers, and although her husband's sexual infidelities don't directly damage her own chances of reproduction, she nevertheless risks one or more of these indiscretions turning into something more enduring, encouraging him to divert his time and resources away from his children by her. And although today women's capacity to support themselves means that the

hildren of single mothers are not automatically jeopardised, for 99 per
ent of our evolutionary history, this was not the case. Unless she had very
xtensive (and very generous) kin, an abandoned prehistoric female may
ave had little chance of keeping her child, or even herself, safe and in a
ood state of health.

Bearing in mind the different priorities of men and women, Daly and
Wilson expected that the triggers for jealousy might be weighted slightly
differently in each sex. Men, they believed, might be aroused to greater
ealousy by the threat of physical infidelity, and women by the sort
f emotional withdrawal that might signal impending desertion and
he reallocation of their partner's resources. Several early studies had
inted that this might be the case. In one, men were shown to react
with anger to jealousy-inducing situations, while women would respond
with either tears, feigned indifference, or attempts to make themselves
more attractive. The results were suggestive, but it wasn't until David Buss
ecame familiar with Daly and Wilson's work, and decided to test it in the
aboratory, that the distinction was made manifest.

Buss knew that he would be on dangerous ground with any sort of
ractical investigation of sexual jealousy. He tells of a researcher in Illinois
who tried to measure sexual jealousy by asking men's wives to speak to
im in a flirtatious fashion. Their husbands were sitting in a next-door
oom, able to hear everything that was going on but unaware that the
irtation was purely experimental. After several trial runs, in which more
han one enraged husband crashed into the laboratory and tried to beat
p the hapless investigator, the project was abandoned.

If he was to gather anything more solid than anecdotal evidence, Buss
eeded to be more careful, more precise. The method he settled on was
o recruit a group of sixty men and women, all in long-term relationships,
nd place them, one by one, in a physiological laboratory where their
rown rates, heartbeats and perspiration levels could be monitored. Each
ubject was asked to imagine two possible scenarios. In the first, their
artner was forming a deep emotional attachment with another person.
n the second, they were enjoying a one-off sexual encounter. There was
 cooling-off period between each scenario, and physiological readings
were taken throughout. Reflecting Buss's expectation perfectly, the women
howed greater physiological responses to the emotional scenario, and
men to the physical one. Indeed, faced with the image of their long-term
artner in bed with another man, the average male heartbeat increased

to a level comparable to that produced by three straight cups of coffee. Jealousy, it seemed, was indeed endemic to both sexes, yet slightly different in each.

But if Daly and Wilson were to demonstrate that jealousy is a truly universal phenomenon, they also had to debunk the idea that certain people, and certain cultures, were free from its effects. It didn't take them long. Picking through the ethnographies of so-called 'jealousy-free' cultures extolled by sociologists, they gathered evidence of the jealous rage of cuckolded husbands in every one – evidence which was not all that hard to find. The very same ethnography which was traditionally cited to prove the absence of jealousy among the Marquesas contains direct references to its existence, and its power. 'When a woman undertook to live with a man, she placed herself under his authority,' it reads. 'If she cohabited with another man without his permission, she was beaten or, if her husband's jealousy was sufficiently aroused, killed.' And when Daly and Wilson looked at reports of life among other societies, the pattern was much the same. Although the Diere practised a system of multiple marriages, in which a woman was sexually available to several men, bloodshed in sexual jealousy disputes was legendary; and among the Hidatsa of North America, although sexual jealousy was reviled, it was an ever-present force. 'Some husbands nearly killed their wives because they went with other men,' confessed one Hidatsa woman.

In all these reports, as with the work concerning sexual jealousy in general, the focus has primarily been on men, not because women are less jealous, but because the jealous rage of men has traditionally been more spectacularly visible and, in societal terms, more deadly. The rage of the cuckolded husband is a staple of folklore and literature, and the jealous instinct stretches right back through history to the formative days of humanity.

Seen in this light, the thousands of incarcerated wife-killers in the West are not all inhuman monsters; they are human beings acting on human impulses, however out of control. But in the past, as today, no culture could benefit in the long run from the struggle caused by men continually competing over each other's wives, and the misery and murder which often followed. While in some circumstances revenge might have felt like a victory, however bitter-sweet, for the husband, it was a disaster for the culture, whose numbers were depleted and whose ranks seethed with violent men and miserable, endangered women. Better by far to institute prevention than have to live with such a drastic and self-defeating cure.

Any society that wished to grow and flourish would have had to devise a structure for human sexual relations which would maximise co-operation and minimise jealous conflict. Of course, it would help if the sexual culture was stuffed with exhortations, hedged round with prohibitions, sanctified by religion and policed by the full force of the law. And so it was that marriage came to be not just the ceremonial coming together of a man and a woman, but the bedrock of the way in which societies have organised themselves throughout history.

Marital law

In the Ancient Near Eastern section of the Musée du Louvre in Paris, a large black obelisk stands proudly on a square stone plinth. Engraved with the wisdom of the ages, and cordoned from public touch by a crimson velvet rope, the obelisk is inscribed with some of the earliest laws in history, dating from 1750 BC. It is the work of Hammurabi, leader of the Babylonian empire, whose territory stretched across the whole of ancient Mesopotamia from the Mediterranean coast of Syria to the shores of the Black Sea.

Hammurabi was an empire-builder in the truest sense of the word, extending his dominion by conquest and enforcing his will by law. Yet he knew that the security of his reign depended on the stability of his people, and so his laws were primarily constructed not to propagandise international conquest but to promote internal stability. To this end, they concerned themselves with three inter-related issues.

First, each man's property was sacrosanct. In the days before settlement, when people had roamed the grasslands of Africa engaging in communal hunting and communal living, this issue had been relatively unimportant. There was little concept of personal ownership because there was little to own, and few differences in wealth. By contrast, in settled civilisations like Hammurabi's, hard labour, brute force or birthright could endow some people with considerable amounts of land to cultivate or personal fortunes to consolidate. The capacity to enjoy them without interference was now crucial. Even more vital was the ability to pass these advantages down to one's offspring. From a genetic point of view, this was a revolution. For the first time in history, parents could invest in their descendants even after their own deaths. As a result, the laws of Hammurabi – and quite possibly several unwritten codes before his – concentrate first on property rights. No fewer than 140 out of the 282 laws concern ownership.

But, as we remember, the ultimate value of ownership was that a man could attract more and better women to bear him more and better children. Thus the creation and protection of children was the second cornerstone of Hammurabi's law. Fertility was not just sacred, but legally protected. If a woman tried to abort her foetus, she was drowned. If she tried to sterilise her husband by crushing his testicles, she was stoned. And if she failed to bear fruit, he had the right to take a slave as a surrogate mother. The wife might even be obliged to find and buy a suitable slave-woman for him.

Yet the effective channelling of resources to the largest number of children was still pointless unless one could be sure that those children were one's own. The only sure way to do this was to see that a woman arrived in the marital home without being pregnant, and to ensure that she never strayed. And thus, contracts came to be drawn up in which men promised women long-term access to their protection and resources in exchange for exclusive rights to their wombs. These contracts, together with their terms and variations, were the third cornerstone of Babylonian law. They were also the template for Babylonian marriage, and for marriage systems the world over.

In the first part of this contract, the prospective husband bestowed wedding gifts on his bride, in return for which he received a dowry from the girl's family. The dowry, however, was not for his personal use, but as a contribution towards the cost of maintaining her and a kind of insurance for the wife. If he divorced her, he was obliged to return the dowry, or what was left of it, intact. If, as often occurred, the wife remained in her father's house after the marriage, the husband was obliged to pay for her upkeep. If he divorced her, or if she divorced him, he had to continue paying for the upkeep of any children resulting from their union.

This part of the deal was relatively equitable and, to all intents and purposes, humane, but the same could not be said of demands made on a woman's chastity or fidelity, either in Babylon or anywhere thereafter. Men were free to roam where they wished, as long as they didn't infringe another man's rights. For women, the course of later history would be very different. The stage was set for the sorry story of man's obsession with virgin brides and faithful wives, a story that has casually embraced both mutilation and murder.

Virgin brides

The easiest and most failsafe way to ensure that a wife was virginal at her wedding day was to marry her off when her record was before, rather than beyond, reproach. In other words, when she was still a child. Muhammad, founder of the Islamic faith, married his favourite wife Aisha when she was only six years old. And in India and Pakistan today, despite the banning of child marriages, families marry at puberty children who have been betrothed since the age of four or five. In Rajasthan in August 1985, 50,000 children were promised to each other in a series of mass betrothals over two days.

Nor is the West innocent of such techniques. Child marriages have been a favoured technique of European and British elites throughout history, where the aristocracy wished to consolidate landholdings and prevent the corruption of their bloodlines before headstrong children were old enough to have a say. The parish records of the city of Chester in the sixteenth century testify to a marriage between John Somerford, aged three, and Jane Brerton, a blushing bride of two. Halfway through the service, the groom began to grizzle and refused to continue with his vows. After several unsuccessful attempts at persuasion, the priest murmured, 'You must speak a little more, and then go play you.' Five minutes later, little John Somerford was the happiest husband in Chester.

Child marriage has been used across the world and throughout history as perhaps the most widespread way of ensuring that women arrived at the alter unencumbered with the child of another man. Yet it was by no means the most extreme measure taken to ensure virginity. That title must go to a far crueller and more sinister practice: female genital mutilation. Although generally called 'female circumcision', the three main types of mutilation are more akin to castration. Even the most limited form, where a large part of the clitoris is amputated, has devastating effects on both body and mind. The rationale for the operation has always been clear: it should ensure female chastity. Far from the ignorance of early Western societies about the clitoris, other cultures had formed very clear ideas about its role and identified it as the seat of all unruly female desire; as such, it was best cut out, they reasoned, in the hope that a girl would never be tempted to risk her virginity or to cheat on her husband once married.

In harsher forms of mutilation, the inner and outer labia as well as the clitoris would be removed. Yet the most extreme method went even further, aiming not just to eliminate sexual desire, but to prevent premarital penetration altogether. This form of mutilation, known as infibulation or 'Pharaonic circumcision', reflecting its supposed roots in ancient Egypt, involved the complete removal of all the external genitalia, and the sewing up of the wound to leave only one tiny hole, the size of a grain of rice, for the flow of urine and menses. The scar tissue formed by the procedure was so hard and inflexible as to prevent any penetration without extreme damage. When women infibulated in this way were married, they would have to be 'opened' with a knife to allow their husbands to penetrate them, and later cut even further to allow for childbirth. Even after such an ordeal, infibulation would be repeated after birth, to guard the woman's chastity between procreative periods.

Female genital mutilation in all its forms is a barbarism not just of the past: across Africa and the Middle East, from Senegal to Oman, over 120 million living women have endured it.

Happily for some, loss of virginity can now be cured as well as prevented. In upper-crust settings, from doctors' surgeries in Harley Street and the plusher districts of Middle Eastern cities to the most prestigious hospitals in Japan, some surgeons have started up a highly profitable sideline in restoring broken hymens. The appearance, if not the reality, of a virgin bride can be produced either by a form of infibulation, stitching together whatever vestiges of a hymen might remain, or more subtly by grafting in pieces of sheep gut to create a second, artificial barrier.

Fumihiko Umezawa of the Jujin Hospital in Tokyo is an expert in the procedure, which in Japan is given the cheerful euphemism 'hymen rebirth'. Although Japanese society has rarely been all that concerned with bridal virginity, his business is still booming. Clients tend to fall into four main categories. First are victims of child abuse or rape, for whom the operation can function as a kind of restorative ritual. Second, there are divorcees from some of Japan's wealthiest families who are about to remarry; in these circles, at least a symbolic show of virginity is considered good form. Third, there are a number of cases of women who have worked in the sex industry but are now engaged; for them, a new hymen signals a fresh start for their husbands and the abandonment of their old way of life.

But by far the largest number of Dr Umezawa's clients are women from richer countries in the Middle East (the Gulf States in particular) who have had premarital sex, and whose reputations, and even lives, would be seriously threatened if their husbands found out they weren't virgins.

In Africa, the Mediterranean and the Middle East, overlapping with local forms of female circumcision, is the equally long-established tradition of sheet showing, in which a groom or female relative is obliged to wave a bloody sheet from the bridal bower to signal the rupturing of the new wife's hymen. In many cases, it's a 'proof' for which the happy couple have often had to thank an aunt, a knife, and a nearby animal rather than the bride's premarital conduct. However, where there is no proof of any kind, the new bride might be publicly shamed, returned to her own kin in disgrace, or even killed for dishonouring the family name. More pragmatic societies could allow a husband cheated of a virgin bride to either return the wife while keeping the dowry, or keep the wife and claim some extra cash damages.

In cultures where virginity was essential, the stakes were far higher. The book of Leviticus prescribes that those ancient Hebrew brides who didn't pass the stained-sheet test should be stoned to death outside the city gates. Most frightening of all, the bride's own family could be pressured to punish and even kill her. Even today, in both Christian and Muslim Arab communities of the Middle East, cases of 'honour killing' regularly crop up. Girls and women who are known to have had, or even just suspected of having had, sex before marriage can be executed with the full knowledge and approval of much of the community. Such killings are usually ignored by the police and under-reported by the media. In a bitter twist, the 'duty' of honour killing often falls to the unfortunate young woman's father or brothers.

Generally, these highly literal forms of proof are being phased out, to be replaced by more symbolic tokens of virginity. Today in the Christian West, virginity is hinted at in the gauzy veil which a bride wears down the aisle, in her crisp, white dress, and in the retention of a nine-month engagement period, during which signs of an unwelcome pregnancy could be spotted and investigated. We've grown accustomed to thinking of these trappings of Western marriage as the hallmarks of romance; but in fact they hark back to a bloody history of fear and punishment.

Faithful wives

The requirements for bridal virginity have been stark and pervasive, but even once a woman had made it to the altar, her troubles were only just beginning. For every technique that had once been employed to ensure her virginity, there was another to enforce her continuing fidelity.

It wasn't enough that a woman had arrived in her husband's home unencumbered with another man's child. Every effort had to be made to ensure that she would never have the chance to cuckold her husband, and thus foist impostors on to his estate. And so the imbalance in the marriage contract, which had been there from the start, began to widen ever further. Men might stray, but women, never.

First, and most blatantly, a husband could physically restrict his wife's movements, forbidding her to leave the house. Any contact with men not from her own or her husband's family was completely banned. This sort of seclusion reached an extreme in Islamic societies, from the inward-looking mud courtyards of northern Nigeria to the elaborately decorated harems of Mogul India. On the eastern coast of Africa, it was a Swahili proverb that a truly virtuous woman left her home only twice in her life: once on the day of her wedding, and again on the day of her funeral. Yet the confinement of women was going on far earlier in human history. The women of ancient Athens, supposedly the cradle of democracy, actually had less freedom of movement than women in the Ayatollah's Iran of the twentieth century: they simply did not go out, even to do the market shopping. Their only leave was to visit women's religious events. The writer Lysias sang the praises of his sister and niece, paragons of Greek female virtue, 'with so much concern for their modesty that they were embarrassed even to be seen by their male relatives'.

Where women were allowed out of the marital home, they might be placed in a sort of mobile seclusion, carried in heavily curtained litters, protected from view by cloth screens wielded by attendants, or shrouded in garments which covered their entire bodies. Heavy veiling, obscuring the outlines of the body and sometimes even the face, sent a clear signal that these women were taken, and not available to any men other than their husbands. Men, as well as women, were exhorted in Islam to be modest, both in dress and behaviour, but women in particular were to avoid flirtatious behaviour and eye contact, 'guarding in secret that which Allah hath guarded'.

From around the eleventh century AD, Chinese society took even more concrete measures to prevent female roving, binding women's feet so that they could hardly walk, let alone run. Starting while a girl was a child and the bones in her feet still malleable, a specialist in footbinding would constrict the feet into tiny, twisted knots and bind them with ever-tighter cloth bands. The toes would be forced right under the sole of the foot and the instep bent double, so the ball almost touched the heel. The overall length of the feet was drastically reduced; the ideal length for upper-class women was a tiny four inches. Each binding was acutely painful, making walking an agony and deforming the foot for ever. Yet bound feet became a requirement of female beauty and a Chinese national fetish, rhapsodised over by poets and sternly assessed by potential mothers-in-law, who would reject out of hand any possible brides with 'big' – that is, normal – feet.

Restrictions on married women were applied all over the world. From the Middle Ages, European women may have had more freedom of movement than their counterparts in China or the Middle East, but their conduct was no less closely monitored. When they did venture outside their husband's house they were usually escorted by either a male guard or an older female companion, who was obliged to repel any intruding males and report back on any misconduct. Where husbands had to leave their wives alone for any length of time, some historians hold that they could physically enforce their chastity by locking them into clanking metal chastity belts, contraptions designed to prevent any possible penetration.

Of course, not all these methods could be universally enforced. In most societies, poor women escaped the strictest forms of seclusion through sheer necessity. They had to go out to work, so all-enveloping veils, palanquins and lives spent behind high walls were simply not an option. In fact, seclusion also began to serve as a mark of social distinction. It soon became a truism that the richer a family was, the more exaggeratedly it would advertise the restriction and reservation of its women. In India, the elite would have narrower windows in its women's quarters; in the Middle East, its women would go out less and less; in Egypt, its daughters would be the most heavily veiled; and in China, only the upper classes could afford to hobble their women by binding their feet.

While physical methods of seclusion and restriction might have soothed the concerns of possessive husbands, they all had drawbacks. Human ingenuity would find a way round any kind of concrete restriction. More

efficient, in the long run, would be mental restrictions, which would
attempt to dissuade women (and intruding males) from ever wanting
to engage in extramarital adventures. The rhetoric employed by family,
religion and law to enforce this might take one of two forms. In the
first, more positive approach, people could be exhorted to fidelity as a
virtue in itself; virginity before marriage and faithfulness after would lead
to family honour, personal reputation, and a good life in the hereafter. But
more effective still was the negative approach, which threatened terrible
punishment for any woman who committed adultery, and any man who
tempted her to do so.

'The wages of sin is death'

Over the course of history, adultery has incurred penalties from a simple
fine to the ultimate punishment – execution. Hammurabi's Code was
blunt and straightforward on this point: adulterous wives and their lovers
were to be tied up and thrown in the river to drown. Classical laws
allowed husbands the right to execute the lovers, although not the wives.
Even today, adultery is a capital offence in six countries – Afghanistan,
Bangladesh, Iran, Pakistan, Somalia and Sudan – with execution usually
by the biblical and straightforwardly brutal method of stoning.

The death penalty for adultery might seem harsh enough in itself, but
the act of extramarital sex has also inspired some of the nastiest and most
ingenious methods of execution in history. It seemed to bring out the most
vicious thirst for revenge, as cultures vied to produce new and ever more
elaborate forms of physical punishment. The Vietnamese used to throw
straying wives to elephants which had been specially trained to toss them
in the air and then trample them to death. The Cheyenne of North
America, the Zulu of southern Africa and the Igbo of what is now Nigeria
would respectively gang-rape adulterous wives, thrust cactus plants into
their vaginas, and tie them to the ground with their lovers, where they
were forced to copulate while stakes were driven through their conjoined
bodies. Even the annals of the supposedly high-minded Romans contain
references to split limbs, castration and forced anal insertion of spiked fish
when it came to adultery.

The very word 'adultery' comes from the Latin *adulterare*, meaning to
admix an alien or inferior substance; we still talk about 'adulterated' food.

In the sexual sphere, this alien substance could be only one thing: the sperm (and hence the genes) of an intruding male. And this term betrays the fundamental sex bias of laws about extramarital sex. For most of history, in fact, adultery has been a sex-specific offence, committed only by married women and their lovers. Married men who had sex with girls or widows were simply not classed as adulterers; so the fearful penalties for adultery fell only on to intruding men and cheating wives.

Wives might be killed, but were just as frequently subjected to more prolonged punishment. Some interpretations of the Quran inspired jurists to decree that adulterous wives should be walled up inside a single room of their husband's house for the rest of their lives. Legends of medieval Europe recount more than one story of knights who, when they discovered their wives' affairs, not only killed the men who had cuckolded them, but then forced the women to drink from the skulls of their dead lovers. While husbands might be restrained from killing their wives by concerns about their children's survival, there was nothing to stop bitter cuckolds from beating, starving and abusing their wives until they died after years of misery.

Intruding male lovers were more likely to be dispatched quickly – even killed on the spot. Husbands who took the law into their own hands have often been exonerated, or even encouraged. Ancient Greek husbands were officially allowed to kill an intruding male with impunity, provided he had committed adultery under the husband's own roof. As late as 1974, section 1225 of the Texas Penal Code allowed that any man who found his wife *in flagrante delicto* with another man could kill him and be guilty of nothing more than justifiable homicide, which wouldn't even result in a trial, much less a punishment. Even where legal codes prescribed some limits on cuckolds' revenge, adultery was always recognised as being second only to mortal fear as a valid reason to kill. Traditions of law following the English system nearly always bring a charge of manslaughter rather than murder against men who kill their wives, or their wives' lovers, after discovering adultery. Following the great English legal commentator Blackstone, the law accepts that, for a reasonable man, 'there can be no greater provocation'.

The traditional allowances made for cuckolds' rage might have been reined in, but they are still very much alive. In August 1997, Lord Justice Prosser followed in the footsteps of Blackstone, causing national outrage by giving a wife-killer no greater penalty than two hundred hours' community service to 'atone' for his wife's death. After hearing welder David Swinburne's account of his wife Margaret's adultery, their turbulent marriage, and his emotional explosion, the judge pronounced that 'No public need would be met by putting you in custody.' Evidently, Swinburne's plea that when his wife told him she was about to abandon him and go to live with her lover, he 'just went crazy', touched the judge's heart.

There was, however, another vital factor in the formulation and enforcement of adultery laws: money. We've already seen how preoccupied Hammurabi's Code, and later legal systems, were with property and status, and how strict seclusion of women was the prerogative of the wealthy. In the rules on adultery, as in most other fields, there was one law for the rich and another for the poor. Males from the high echelons of all societies were unlikely to suffer any penalties at all for forcing their sexual attentions on poorer men's wives. But if low-status men cuckolded those at the top, they could expect to have the book thrown at them. The more the resources at stake, the more horrible the punishment suffered by an intruding male. Among the Ashanti of Ghana, for example, adultery with a commoner's wife was a private matter and incurred a simple monetary fine. Sleeping with the wife of a chief, by contrast, condemned a man to an agonising, long-drawn out death by a hundred cuts from a machete, in front of the entire community.

Polygamy to monogamy

Throughout history, in matters of marriage and fidelity, the jealousy of proprietary husbands was matched only by the envy of the proletariat. The institution of marriage, as we've seen, was often more about property and inheritance than individual commitment. The majority of human societies allowed men of the elite to marry as many women as they could support, and often to take numerous concubines as well, but wherever societies allowed richer men to accumulate women unchecked, social unrest soon followed. In polygamous societies, where men could marry and monopolise all the women they could afford, there would inevitably be a pool of men at the bottom of the heap who had little or no chance of having a wife and children of their own. The perennial tension between haves and have-nots was only worsened by the concentration of fertile women around the men of the elite. Being lorded over by a richer man was bad enough, but being denied even the chance of sex was an even greater provocation.

Some tribal cultures, like the Yanomamo and certain Aboriginal groups, tried to get round the problem by marrying off girls as young as possible, sometimes reserving them as future wives of the chief even before they were born. In these same societies, young men might have to wait until their thirties or even forties before they would have a chance to marry. Larger, more centralised groups and empires, where the top dogs had accumulated vast harems, thus making the sexual prospects of poor men even gloomier, had to resort to more ruthless measures. Few things were as dangerous to the good order of a sophisticated society as a huge, seething mass of sexually frustrated, unmarried young men. The despotic rulers and powerful chiefs of polygamous societies had to resort to ingenious and ruthless methods to keep the lid on. Often, the best available solution was to conscript young males into the army and pack them off to war, thereby preventing them from causing unrest at home and possibly giving them an opportunity to capture a wife of their own. Vast numbers of men could be sent into exhausting and often fatal industries like mining or sailing.

But all these measures were essentially stopgaps. They couldn't work for long because they failed to address the basic problem. Polygamy worsened sexual jealousy and competition between men, rendering society as a whole less stable. If the situation was to be resolved, the rulers of such societies were going to have to stop hogging the women and buy loyalty from men in the lower ranks by devolving wives to them.

The Inca empire, whose rulers accumulated staggering numbers of concubines, was careful to reward its barons and generals with impressive sexual opportunities. By doling out the cast-offs from the emperor's harem, which tended not to keep women on once they had passed the age of thirty, and formulating a complex sliding scale of tribute, the Incas hedged their bets and made sure their well-ordered, delicately balanced society stayed afloat. While the emperor's household could contain thousands of women and the lords of the kingdom could claim up to four hundred concubines, chiefs and 'principal persons' were allotted fifty each, 'so that there might be more people in the kingdom'. Leaders of vassal nations were given twenty women, mid-level administrators twelve, minor chieftains eight and village headmen anything from seven to three, depending on the number of men they commanded.

And the Incas were not alone, for running unnoticed beneath the entire sweep of history, as it moves on from the age of the despots, through more modified power in early modern societies to the upheavals of industrial revolution and eventual democracy, is a little-noticed sexual transition. And this private, personal transition mirrors our official, public history in an intriguing way. Just as power has been gradually devolved, so have been women. Again and again, in different societies and in different places, societies which once tolerated polygamy have quietly switched strategies and instituted monogamous marriage – one woman for one man. It's a transition which strikes some commentators as a mere coincidence because, they argue, the move to monogamy has occurred at so many disparate points in history that there can be no common cause for the switch.

Laura Betzig, who knows more than most about the workings of harems and despots, begs to differ. She is quite definite that socially enforced monogamy, tying a man, however rich he may be, to one spouse at a time, is the historical exception. In her view, it's a phenomenon with clearly identifiable causes. Having a system of one-man-one-wife, she argues, is directly related to a political system of one-man-one-vote. Where democracy takes root, men will naturally vote themselves wives, limiting the ambitions of despots sexually as well as politically. And where ideas about individual freedoms really take off, they have often been fuelled by other spurs to monogamy: monotheistic religion (one man, one God), literacy and, most crucially, mobility. The slaves of ancient Greece or Rome, or even the peasants of medieval Europe, had little choice but to stay put and tolerate their masters' harems. Once it became possible to get up and leave – to a larger town, to a city, or even a new continent – polygamy tended to die out. Poor men voted with their feet.

Polygamy isn't *inherently* any less stable than monogamy. In many circumstances, it has proved the quickest way for small societies to go forth and multiply, with their strongest men dominating sexually as well as socially. From the patriarchs of the ancient Hebrews to the strongmen of the Yanomamo and the emperors of China, polygamous men have made history. But the rumbling desires of the poorer and now forgotten men have shaped its course just as decisively. The underdog really has won out in the end. We find today that, although the majority of the world's *societies* allow polygamy, with less than a fifth of all known cultures insisting on monogamy, the vast majority of the world's *people* are, and always have been, monogamous. And as Western influence has spread around the world, either through choice or by force, the move to monogamy has spread with it. Polygamy is not dead. In some parts of the world it's alive and well, and looks set to continue for some time. But in the long run, seen in historical perspective, it's on the way out.

Conclusion

In this chapter I've attempted, like Theseus picking his way through the maze, to travel through the global history and culture of sex, hanging on to some vital basic threads. Beneath the colourful and varied tapestry of different cultures, three principal concerns emerge. First, and so basic it often goes unnoticed, lies the fundamental concern of most human beings, male and female, to survive and to pass on their genes. Later come incest and marriage, the interlocking twin obsessions of human society, which become the focus of immense cultural effort. To survive and prosper, the earliest human groups had to find a way to avoid incest. The solution, of sending women to men in neighbouring groups, was the origin of the concept of marriage, crystallising ideas of property and exchange which would be fundamental to group living from then on.

Yet marriage was destined to create as many problems as it solved; problems of jealousy and violence which became exacerbated when people settled into communities and adopted the idea of ownership. There were now estates to be handled, fortunes to be made, and goods to be handed on, and if tribes were to grow into stable cultures, they needed to make sure that those gods went to legitimate heirs.

Women, all too often the pawns in the marriage contract, now became subject to fierce restrictions, their fertility monitored and their movements curtailed. Then, as cultures grew ever more sophisticated, a fissure emerged between those who had much power and many women and those who had little and few. At first, women were heavily stockpiled and strictly guarded, with ever more elaborate contraptions to hem them in, but eventually, as leaders recognised that their power depended as much on the men they ruled as on the goods they amassed, they began to devolve their women until, eventually, monogamy – and democracy – became the order of the day.

This picture of the emergence and growth of human culture is a far cry from that advanced by sociologists and historians only a few decades ago. For whereas in more traditional schemas, sex has been seen as little more than a quirky footnote in the history of humankind, here it is placed at the very centre, as the organising principle and fundamental concern of societies the world over; as the source of society itself. But while this rule applies very generally across the human species, individual cultures were grappling with widely varying conditions. To keep afloat from day to day, they had to institute their own particular rules about outbreeding, marriage and fidelity in very particular ways. For all the common underlying threads, human sexual behaviour has never been the same everywhere in the world. Different conditions have led to local, more specific variations on the basic themes. Each culture has had to make its own rules – and those rules could have a radical, even bizarre, effect on the sexuality of its citizens.

The next chapter looks in some detail at the sexuality of the West.

4

The Christian Heritage

On Wednesday, 26 March 1997, the San Diego County Communication Center logged the following telephone call:

CALLER: Hello?
OPERATOR: Hello.
CALLER: I need to report an anonymous tip. Who do I talk to?
OPERATOR: Okay. This is regarding what?
CALLER: This is regarding a mass suicide.

Two minutes later Lieutenant G. Lipscomb was in his squad car headed for 18241 Collina Norte in the Rancho Santa Fe district. As he swept into the driveway, he could see the muslin curtains billowing through a dozen open windows. He stepped out of the car and entered gingerly through the back door. What he saw amazed him. Lying prostrate on the beds, the sofas, and all along the corridors were thirty-nine bodies, each fully clothed, their arms extended by their sides, their feet placed neatly together. Over each of their faces, a square of purple cloth had been placed. The bodies looked peaceful; purposeful, even. As if they knew where they were going.

It soon emerged that they did. After being told of the mass suicide, the police had been given a copy of a videotape. Made by the people among whose bodies Lipscomb had been walking, it revealed that they were members of a radical religious cult called Heaven's Gate, whose members believed that they had come from outer space, that they had been put on Earth as souls to grow and be harvested, and that the comet Hale-Bopp was now summoning them back to heaven before the planet was engulfed in disaster and destruction. Once in heaven, the cult members would ascend to the 'level above human', in which emotion was annihilated, gender dissolved and sex banished; a state which many had attempted to emulate on Earth by abandoning sex-specific clothing, adopting chastity and (in the case of eight of the men) by castrating themselves.

Heaven's Gate was the latest in a long line of breakaway religious cults to emerge in a time of profound cultural uncertainty, and which were designed to appeal to the poor (by advocating the supremacy of spiritual over material wealth), to the downtrodden (by positing a better life in the hereafter), and to the directionless (by offering a clear, if unorthodox, path to salvation).

Although their charismatic leader, Marshall Applewhite, chose the Internet as his preaching platform and used a vernacular all his own, the claims made by Heaven's Gate and the effects it had on its followers were remarkably similar to those of another breakaway sect, which had started in a not dissimilar way nearly two thousand years ago. The difference is that one, thankfully, was a drop in the ocean, while the other has shaped the sexuality of half the world.

Prophet in a melting pot

It all started so well. In the first century BC, most of the Western world was a fiercely patriarchal place, dominated by the Roman Empire and still drawing on the wisdom of the great Greek culture which had preceded it. Both cultures operated a nominally monogamous marriage system, but both also allowed men almost total leeway to expand their repertoire of sexual partners beyond the marital bed. For the rich at least, this meant frequent congress with slaves, concubines, prostitutes and teenage boys. The lot of women, however, was not so happy. In Greece, married women were confined to their own section of the house, rarely took part in public activities, and spent their lives subject to male authority, whether that of a father, a husband or a son. In Rome, while wives were nominally better off (possessing, for instance, the right of divorce), they continued to be passed as property from their fathers to their husbands, to be treated by the former as a valuable bargaining chip to secure wealth and real estate, and by the latter as a mobile womb.

Set against this, in the Middle Eastern lands around Palestine, was the equally male-dominated and expansionist Jewish culture, obsessed with racial purity but insistent on multiplying its numbers so that it would be physically capable of populating the lands it had been promised. To this end, much of Jewish law was promulgated to ensure that women bore children to their husbands and to their husbands only, and that they bore as many children as possible. Women who were barren could be divorced out of hand; those caught in the act of adultery could be hunted down and stoned to death.

On the face of it the Jewish sexual regime, like those of the Romans and Greeks, seemed generally positive about sex, and indeed went to some lengths to promote it. Polygamy was actively encouraged, provided that the husband aimed at procreating with as many of his wives as possible; concubinage was common; and the most sagacious rabbis set their minds to specifying targets for sexual congress that all good Jews should aim to achieve: once a night for gentlemen of leisure, twice a week for labourers, once a week for donkey drivers and twice a year for sailors. But the flip side of these exhortations was a fierce denunciation of all non-procreative sexual acts. For men, homosexuality was considered anathema, bodily fluids were polluting, and sex with beasts was energetically denounced. But, as we have seen, the full force of the Jewish emphasis on procreation fell on women.

By the first century BC, the Romans had extended their empire to incorporate much of the eastern Mediterranean, including the Jewish homeland of Judaea. As a result, it was into this cultural melting-pot, seething with racial tensions, shot through with chauvinism and bent on procreation, that Jesus of Nazareth was born in Bethlehem of Judaea some time between 7 and 4 BC.

Jesus

By the earliest and most reliable account of his life, given in the Gospel according to St Mark, we have no reason to believe that Jesus' birth was marked in any special way. His father, Joseph, was an observant Jew who traced his lineage back to the time of David; his mother, an ordinary if devout woman. Jesus himself, who appears to have had brothers and sisters (though it is not clear how many), grew up in the small village of Nazareth, set among the hills above Galilee, and looked set to follow his father into the carpentry trade.

It was not until he was about twelve that there appeared to be something unusual about the boy. He had read the scriptures, as had most children of his age, but he also seemed to have assimilated them to an extraordinarily high degree – so much so that, on a visit to Jerusalem, his mother found him surrounded by the scribes of the temple, holding forth on complex issues of rite and meaning. A few years later, during his late teens or early twenties, Jesus left home and travelled south to Bethany, where he was baptised in the River Jordan by his cousin John, who would later become one of his most ardent supporters. He then retreated to the desert, where legend has it he was tempted by Satan, before gathering a following of twelve trusted disciples and returning to Galilee to preach. Unfortunately, neither the Jews nor the Romans much liked what they heard.

Jesus' primary message was extremely simple and best summed up in the words attributed to him by Mark during a visit to Jerusalem: 'Thou shalt love the Lord thy God with all thy heart, and with all thy soul, and with all thy mind, and with all thy strength . . . And thou shalt love thy neighbour as thyself.' This two pronged devotion, both to God and to the well-being of others, was very much in line with traditional Jewish thought. But although the words were orthodox, it soon became clear that Jesus' interpretation of them was not.

By preaching that the kingdom of God could, and soon would, be found on Earth, Jesus appeared to challenge the authority of the Romans. By overturning the tables of the money-changers in the temple and suggesting that God was most effectively worshipped free of charge, he angered the Jews. But most surprising of all, in a move which was inflammatory to Jews and Romans alike, his understanding of the phrase 'love thy neighbour as thyself' seemed to include women as well as men.

When a group of scribes seized a woman who had been caught in the act of adultery and brought her to Jesus, asking him what he thought of their plan to stone her, Jesus paused, and then suggested that whoever was without sin should cast the first stone. Later, when preaching that the kingdom of God was at hand, he made a special point of including even the most despised sector of Jewish society, barren women. But it was his stand on divorce which occasioned then, as for centuries to come, the most heated debate.

The rabbis and the Romans, as we have seen, taught that wives should make good housekeepers and good mothers. If they did, fine; if not, they should be abandoned without much ceremony. The only disagreement was about how many misdemeanours should be overlooked. Some rabbis argued that everything short of adultery should be pardoned; others, that even the most minor fall from grace was sufficient to occasion dismissal. Thus, according to Rabbi Hillel, a man should be able to leave his wife 'even if she burns the soup'.

While he was preaching on the far side of the river Jordan, Jesus was approached by a group of learned Jews and asked for his views on exactly this question: 'Is it lawful for a man to put away his wife?' As so often, he first parried their question with another: 'What did Moses command you?'

'Moses suffered to write a bill of divorcement, and to put her away.'

Then came the shocker.

'For the hardness of your heart he wrote you this precept. But from the beginning of the creation, God made them male and female. For this cause shall a man leave his father and mother, and cleave to his wife. What therefore God has put together, let not man put asunder.'

The sonorous tone of this proclamation, as well as its revolutionary content, was met with stony silence before the Jews filed slowly away. No one could quite believe their ears. Shortly afterwards, even Jesus' disciples asked him whether he was sure about what he had been saying. Jesus was adamant. 'Whosoever shall put away his wife, and marry another, commiteth adultery against her. And if a woman shall put away her husband, and be married to another, she commiteth adultery.'

The idea that marriage was a lifelong bond for the husband as for the wife, and could be dissolved neither on grounds of adultery nor infertility, was anathema to two cultures both bent on procreation, and a first in the history of the world.

In a roundabout and rather ironic way, Jesus' revolutionary message functioned as one of the world's earliest feminist manifestos. Following his preaching, a new hope must have arisen for women. Marriage might not be the most comfortable or egalitarian sexual arrangement in the world, but if it were necessary for the peaceful continuation of the species, making it indissoluble certainly evened out the sexual stakes a little. Women could expect more clement treatment from the law (if not from their husbands), a renewed emphasis on the companionate nature

of marriage, and a less paranoid concern over the function and fruitfulness
of their wombs. Jesus' own life, marked by enduring friendships and
possibly even devoid of sex, was a further endorsement of this, as was
his praise of John the Baptist's celibacy. In an age when priests, above
all, were expected to create an example to their followers by obeying
God's command to 'be fruitful and multiply', this was a revolutionary
message indeed.

Unfortunately, Jesus' last days were marked by a growing vengefulness
on the part of the Jewish authorities, and by intimations of immortality
from Jesus himself. Finally, when he rode triumphantly into Jerusalem on
the back of a donkey, he was arrested, tried for overstepping the mark,
and taken to Golgotha to be crucified.

This might have signalled an abrupt and inglorious end to yet another
marginal prophet, but his execution in fact signalled a new and extraordinary dawn. By the time Jesus died, he had gathered around him such a
devoted and energetic following that neither his name nor his message
would be eclipsed. The position of women, one might hope, was about
to be elevated and the obsession with sex quelled. Pity would be taken on
the poor, the helpless, and the needy. People everywhere might lead more
peaceful, equitable, productive lives, free from persecution and shame.

This, at least, is what should have happened. But it was not to be.

In the early centuries after Jesus' death, there emerged in the deserts
of Jordan and the provinces of the Near East a number of extraordinary
preachers who would see, in the name of Jesus, rather different possibilities. Blessed with less pure lives and less noble purposes, they were
about to hijack his teachings and turn them into a wholesale programme
for the subscription and manipulation of millions of disaffected souls in
the twilight years of the Roman Empire. Instead of clemency, they would
preach judgement. Instead of mercy, hellfire. Instead of the kingdom of
heaven on earth, imminent apocalypse or a complete rejection of earthly
concerns. They were, of course, Paul, Jerome and Augustine; the unholy
trinity of early Christianity and the first great spin-doctors of the nascent
Christian faith.

Lives of the spin-doctors

'This man has introduced a new teaching, bizarre and disruptive of the human race. He denigrates marriage: yes, marriage, which you might say is the beginning, root, and fountainhead of our nature.'

The speaker, in this fifth-century account of the life of St Thecla, is Thamyris, a prosperous young man who was to have been Thecla's husband. The villain he is denouncing for leading his fiancée to abandon him for a life of virginity is none other than St Paul, whose passionate rhetoric and fierce promotion of lifelong chastity would in time frustrate many other planned marriages. This extraordinary man, small, bald and bandy-legged, with a long nose and eyebrows meeting in the middle, was to have an explosive impact on the early Christian faith. His letters to inhabitants around the Mediterranean were so influential that they found their way into the New Testament, and his teachings were so transformative that some suggest Christianity should more accurately be called Paulianity.

Paul was born in the Silician city of Tarsus, near what is now the southern coast of Turkey, in the early years of the first century AD and was brought up as a Greek-speaking Jew with a profound hatred of the faith he would soon adopt. According to the Acts of the Apostles, he spent much of his early life 'breathing out threatenings and slaughter against the Disciples of the Lord', and we have reason to believe he also practised what he preached, consenting to the stoning of the first Christian martyr, Stephen, and seeking permission from the Jewish authorities to hunt down heretics wherever he should find them.

It was on just such a mission, to the ancient and cosmopolitan city of Damascus, that he was suddenly converted. As a man who did nothing by half-measures, Paul was not turned by subtle persuasion, but by a direct and blinding vision of Jesus. The Acts of the Apostles tells us: 'And as he journeyed, he came near Damascus: and suddenly there shined round about him a light from heaven. And he fell to the earth, and heard a voice saying unto him, Saul, Saul, why persecutest thou me? . . . And he trembling and astonished said, Lord, what wilt thou have me do?'

Paul's mission, of course, was to preach the Gospel, a task he performed with the same zeal he had once summoned to decry it. Unfortunately, he wasn't interested in assimilating the Christian faith as understood by his new colleagues. He was in a hurry, he had received a direct mandate from Jesus, and Jesus, surely, would instruct him in person.

Paul certainly listened to the voices inside his head, but instead of the still, clear tones of Jesus, he heard a crude and discordant medley of the competing philosophies of the Roman Mediterranean. In such a maelstrom of influences, it was perhaps not surprising that his preaching embraced a personal and eclectic mix of Christian mercy, Greek Neo-Platonism and Hebrew procreationism which would betray as much about his past life as about his current calling.

Like Jesus, Paul praised the chaste and the barren but, unlike Jesus, he didn't raise them on to the same level as the married and the childbearing, but on to a pedestal of holiness which far outreached them. To justify his reasoning, he yoked the teachings of Jesus to the Neo-Platonist doctrine of dualism, which taught that the soul was the noblest essence of humanity, trapped in the perishable carcass of the body, and that to abjure earthly pleasures in favour of spiritual contemplation was the path to ultimate fulfilment.

Luckily, despite this message, Paul was a little more realistic than those who would follow, recognising that total abstinence was not a viable option for most. Believing that the second coming was imminent and determined to gather round him as many souls as possible, he was aware that he had to make some concessions to earthly concerns. In his famous first letter to the Corinthians, which has formed the bedrock of Christian thinking on matters of sex and marriage ever since, he thus backtracked a little and suggested that, although marriage was an inferior state to celibacy, it should nevertheless be considered a valid option for Christians, since 'it is better to marry than to burn with desire'.

However, in a further mollifying gesture to Jewish norms, Paul was adamant that sexual life could go no further than this, for when Jesus returned to gather the faithful to his bosom, homosexuals, masturbators and adulterers should go to the back of the queue. 'Be not deceived,' he warned the Corinthians, 'neither fornicators, nor idolaters, nor adulterers, nor effeminate, nor abusers of themselves with mankind . . . shall inherit the kingdom of God.'

Within the space of two decades, Paul had obliterated Jesus' message of tolerance and started to design a pyramid of ascending holiness based on sexual renunciation. This league table of purity would characterise the Christian faith and profoundly affect its followers for nearly two millennia. But if Paul was the conceptual architect of this pyramid, the man who did most to lay its foundations in the real world was Jerome.

During all the time that Paul had been preaching, Christianity was an underground sect promoting a lifestyle that both the Jews and the

Romans hated. Indeed, during the first, second and third centuries AD, many thousands were dragged to the arenas and fed to the lions. But in AD 324, Christianity suddenly became the state religion of the Roman Empire. The emperor Constantine, scared that he was about to lose a battle against his rival Maxentius, swore that if he carried the day he would convert to Christianity. He did both, and the course of Western history was for ever altered.

It was in this atmosphere of new respectability that a young man called Jerome started preaching. Jerome was well aware of the pulling power that the arena had had. On one level, it was horrifying, but on another it had made for fantastic publicity. The Christian martyrs' stoicism in the face of death, and their apparent immunity to pain, had won them a far greater number of converts in the stands than they were losing in the ring.

The athletes for God

With this in mind, Jerome set about reinvigorating the Christian faith with a new ethic, exchanging torture by others for self-inflicted torture. For the new enemy was not the Roman state or the lions in the arena, but internal passions, in particular the state of lust; just as potent, just as hateful, just as destructive. And so began the era of the Desert Fathers: fanatical recluses, both male and female, who abjured all earthly ties and fled to the deserts, where they vied to outdo each other with feats of physical and sexual self-denial.

Some, like the members of Heaven's Gate two millennia later, castrated themselves to be rid of the desire that burned in their loins; others took a different route, deliberately surrounding themselves with nubile women the better to test their powers of resistance. This technique proved so popular that it was still practised as late as the ninth century AD, when the great Irish sage St Swithin was challenged by a fellow monk, St Brendan, over his habit of taking two young virgins to bed. Swithin threw the challenge back at Brendan, who felt himself obliged to do the same. Apparently, Brendan managed to leave his virgins untouched, though he later confessed that he had been unable to sleep all night.

Perhaps the most spectacular of the earlier 'Athletes for God', as they styled themselves, was Simon Stylites, who attacked not just his own lust but the body in which it dwelt. Stylites is most famous for having spent thirty years on top of a sixty-foot pillar. What is less well-known (though equally true) is that he also tied a rope so tightly round his waist that his flesh began to suppurate and swarm with maggots. When these dropped off, Stylites would retrieve them and place them back in his wounds, commanding them to 'Eat what God has given you.'

Jerome, though never the most extreme of the desert-dwellers, was nevertheless their most vocal mouthpiece, commenting frequently on the deviousness and potency of the enemy they were now fighting, and advertising the struggle with scarcely concealed glee. Here, he describes his own sufferings of AD 375:

> Sackcloth disfigured my misshapen limbs, and my skin had become by neglect as black as an Ethiopian's . . . Yet I, who from fear of Hell had consigned myself to that prison where I had no other companions but scorpions and wild beasts, fancied myself among bevies of dancing maidens. My face was pale and my frame chilled with fasting; yet my mind was burning with the cravings of desire, and the fires of lust flared up from my flesh that was as that of a corpse. So, helpless, I used to lie at the feet of Christ, watering them with my tears, wiping them with my hair, struggling to subdue my rebellious flesh.

Here was a powerful enemy indeed. The more one fought against lust, it seemed, the more it returned to haunt one. The more one denied it, the more deeply it dug in its claws. If, under Paul, lust had been seen as a natural force which needed controlling, under Jerome it had become an evil which needed to be resisted. And the greater the resistance, the greater the reward in heaven. It was with this bleak yet ingenious message that Jerome finally left the desert and travelled to Rome, where he immediately zeroed in on that sector of society whom he believed he could most easily convert and most enjoyably resist: the young, aristocratic women of Rome.

Here, he operated as a kind of Rasputin for the chaste, luring his followers into a life of self-denial with his mesmerising personality and intensely seductive prose.

Typically, he would start by denigrating the state of marriage and playing on women's real and well-justified fear of pregnancy and childbirth. 'I praise marriage,' he wrote to one of his followers in 384, 'but only because it gives me virgins. I gather roses from the thorns, the gold from the earth, the pearl from the shell.' But what was in store for those virgins? A life of misery and loneliness, devoid of human affection? Not a bit. Those who abjured the pleasures of the flesh would gain access, in Jerome's scheme of things, to a purer, more mysterious, more all-encompassing eroticism: the eroticism offered by the holy Bridegroom, Jesus. Writing to his young female follower Eustochium, he counselled: 'Let the seclusion of your own chamber ever guard you; ever let the Bridegroom sport within you. If you pray, you are speaking to your Spouse: if you read, He is speaking to you. When sleep falls on you, He will come behind the wall and will put His hand through the hole in the door and will touch your belly. And you will awake and rise up and cry: "I am sick with love."'

This extraordinary framework for worship, in which Christianity punished erotic feelings yet presented itself in candidly erotic terms, would become a key part of its appeal and power in later years. But before it could use this power to bring all good Christians trembling to their knees, it first had to go beyond Paul's pyramid of sexual renunciation, and beyond Jerome's blanket condemnation of all states except virginity, to a world-view in which sex was seen to have sullied and stained the entire human race, from cradle to grave, from the Beginning to the hereafter. This practically superhuman task was to fall to a young bishop from Algeria: St Augustine.

Original sins

Born in AD 354, a decade or so after Jerome, Augustine had an unhappy childhood. His mother, Monica, was a devout Christian, and his father, Patricius, a philandering pagan who cared little for her self-denying ways. These two opposing temperaments would do battle for Augustine's soul over the first three decades of his life, and their clash was never more clearly expressed than in his famous supplication, 'God, give me chastity, but not yet.' As a teenager, he erred towards the fleshly, 'boiling over in [his] fornications', yet even then, he felt the pull of the ascetic life, settling down with a single concubine from the age of seventeen and gravitating slowly towards the hyper-ascetic Manichean sect, who taught that all corporeal concerns, from eating and drinking through to sex, were creations of the Kingdom of Darkness.

In the summer of 386, when he was thirty-two, Augustine was sittin
in his garden one day (pondering the schism between the fleshly and th
spiritual) when he was suddenly seized by a fit of weeping and, lookin
up, heard a childlike voice saying, 'Take up and read; take up and read
He seized the book nearest at hand, a collection of the writings of St Pau
and was converted to Christianity on the spot; a result which delighted hi
mother.

As a newly declared celibate, Augustine took up the baton of Christia
anti-sexualism with all the vigour of the fresh convert. Like so man
preachers and teachers before him, he wrote of the horrific entrapmen
of the soul within the body. But unlike many of them, he knew exactl
whereof he spoke. Augustine's rackety early life had left him all too awar
of the enslaving power of sex. 'It is the keenest of all pleasures on the leve
of sensation,' he wrote (a thought which must have proved tantalisin
for many a celibate novice), '. . . at the crisis of excitement, it practicall
paralyses the power of deliberate thought.'

How could this disobedient flesh, which was capable of overriding th
cool and rational mind, find a proper place in a world created by a
all-powerful and ultimately beneficent God? This was the question t
which Augustine chiefly addressed himself, and his answer would becom
as pernicious as it was preposterous.

He began by proposing that lust had not been part of God's origina
blueprint for the human race. In the garden of Eden, he fantasised, Adar
and Eve would surely have engaged in sex infrequently, dispassionatel
and solely for the procreation of children. The technique they might hav
used was to place Adam's unexcited penis at the opening of Eve's vagina
with ejaculation occurring through an effort of will, of the kind used b
'individuals who can make musical notes issue from the rear of thei
anatomy, so that you would think they were singing'.

Unfortunately, things had not gone quite according to plan. When Ev
ate the apple, she introduced the raging, uncontrollable beast of lust int
the world, which would usurp the once innocent body, 'defying the powe
of will and tyrannising the human sexual organs'. According to thi
schema, lust was not a natural part of creation but a disease introduce
into human nature at the moment of the Fall, responsible for the expulsio
from Eden and staining every generation from that day to this.

Henceforth, the genitals would be recast as pudenda (meaning parts t
be ashamed of), all humans would be born into sin, and every act of se

(involving, necessarily, some element of lust) would bear the imprimatur of man's first and greatest disobedience to God. But that was not all. Since death, too, had followed the Fall, Augustine decided to lump the two together, making lust the cause not just of human frailty but of human mortality as well.

Here was the high water mark of Christian hostility to sex. Never again would Christians live in innocence (even if they were virgins); never again would even married couples make love without the dim sensation that they were doing something wrong, and never again would sex motivated by pleasure rather than procreation (be it heterosexual, homosexual or masturbatory) have any real or valid place in the holy Christian hierarchy.

Between them, in little more than three hundred years, Paul, Jerome and Augustine had changed sexuality in the West more than any other thinkers in the ten millennia which had preceded their ministry or in the two which have so far followed. The pyramid of anti-sexualism which they had so swiftly yet surely constructed had turned sex (during the course of their combined lives) from being the wellspring of human joy to becoming the source of human misery; and from the surest guarantee of immortality into the very origin of death. Indeed, Augustine had managed to recast both sex and death — once the basic and universal facts of nature — as two profoundly unnatural phenomena, and the most obvious signs of humankind's division from God.

The transfiguration of women

Most ironic of all, the teachings of these three men contrived to show that this terrible division, caused by the innate and almost insurmountable sinfulness of human beings, was the fault of women. Women, the sector of society whom Jesus had been so anxious to protect, were now seen as society's chief enemies. Where once the Fall had been perceived as a tragedy of human wilfulness, it was now rewritten as a specifically sexual offence, and one in which woman had sided with the forces of evil. Referring to Eve, who had apparently catalysed the Fall by first tempting Adam, and to Mary, who had somehow managed to transcend the female state by giving birth to Jesus, Augustine writes, 'Through a woman we were sent to destruction, yet through a woman we shall be redeemed.' With this one sentence, he set the tone for the resurrection of the Classical world's traditional antipathy towards women and for an enduring schizophrenia about women's sexuality, whose legacy has still not left us.

Once Paul, Jerome and Augustine had made their feelings about virginity clear, it became all the more essential to emphasise that Jesus himself had been born untainted by sin. In a kind of retrospective clean-up operation, it was stressed that not only had he himself been a virgin but that his mother had too. From being an apocryphal folk-tale, the idea of Mary's virginity became a central pillar of the Christian faith. As the centuries wore on and the volumes of Christian debate and commentary piled up, the myth of Mary's virginity became ever more elaborate and extraordinary. By the early Middle Ages, it was decreed that Mary was not only a virgin before Christ's birth, but had remained intact even during delivery, and then for the rest of her life, with Christ's possible siblings being unceremoniously written out of the picture. At one point, it was even suggested that Mary must have been impregnated not through her vagina but via her ear. Moreover, her physical purity was so incorruptible, it was claimed, that her body didn't deteriorate even after death, and so she was physically received directly into Heaven. She never had menstrual periods and was spared all the pains of childbirth. In short, she wasn't really a flesh-and-blood woman at all.

The cult of Mary, like the Christian religion as a whole, acted as a double-edged sword for women. Initially so promising, giving women a chance to express their own spirituality and take on some of the new spiritual authority, it ended up repressing and condemning most of womankind. The general attitude to women in the early Christian world was as mistrustful and biased as ever. Numerous cults maintained that while men were the Devil's creations below the waist, the entire body of a woman was tainted. The Church itself had only managed to dissolve its fundamental doubts about women in Mary's case by removing from her all those messy, polluting and disturbing attributes of women at large. And while the worship and adoration of Mary might have given women a role model to aspire to, it was a role which would remain forever out of reach for any mortal female. Even the most devout Christian women, from the martyrs of Rome to Jerome's adoring protégées, were never allowed to forget their inferior status.

It's a strange feeling to realise that we should have chosen to canonise

e very men who have most comprehensively damned us. And no more
mfortable to understand that, in many cases, their teachings were
otivated more by their guilt and confusion about their own desires
an by true spiritual calling. However, with the death of Augustine, the
rtain was now falling on the first Act of Christian sexuality; and while
s baleful spirit would hover over all discussions of sex for centuries to
me, the tone in later Acts would often shift from tragedy to farce.

The bishops in the bedroom

hn stood naked in front of the bishop, his clothes in a heap nearby.
e bishop cast an eye over his penis, taking into account its length and
nsistency, then turned and nodded to a woman who sat by the fire.
e woman raised herself to her feet, removed her gown, and checked
e temperature of her hands. They were warm and soft. Slowly, she
proached John, pausing when she was only a foot away to let him
mire her breasts. At a signal from the bishop, she then began her
ork, taking John's penis in her hands and starting to manipulate it.
ter a few moments, the bishop commanded her to stop and show him
e results. John's penis was still flaccid. The bishop nodded again and the
oman returned to her work, this time whispering into John's ear as she
ok his penis in one hand and his testicles in the other. She was clearly
asturbating him. After a few more minutes, she stopped again and John's
nis, once more, was displayed. With holy disdain, the bishop observed
length and circumference. There was no change. He nodded a final time
d the woman went back to work, rubbing furiously on John's penis,
asping his body to hers, smothering him in kisses, and admonishing
m to abandon his reserve and show her his virility. All the while, John
mained motionless and impassive, his face frozen, a faraway look in
s eyes.

Everyone was now staring. Not just the woman and the bishop, but
eryone who had gathered in the room. There was John's brother. His
ends. Sundry witnesses were present too. For this was not a scene
ayed out for the private titillation of the clergy; it was a public divorce
aring (as it happens, in thirteenth-century Canterbury) in which the
aintiff was John's wife, and the issue at stake, his ability to consummate
eir marriage.

A thousand years have passed since the death of Augustine, and in Europe, as in Christendom as a whole, much has happened. Rome has been sacked, the Dark Ages have descended and then lifted, America has been discovered (by the Vikings), and the Eastern and Western Churches have gone their separate ways. Slowly and steadily, the new faith has marched across the world. The Franks are converted in AD 497, the Bulgars and Serbians in 865, and by the end of the eleventh century there is a single church for the whole of Western Christendom, ruled by the Pope in Rome and extending across the entire continent of Europe from Iceland to Italy, and from Sweden to Spain.

While Augustine and his contemporaries had lured millions into the Christian way of life by skilfully counterpointing the Romano-Jewish obsession with procreation, the church of the medieval period sought to keep its converts Christian by imposing a strict and logical code of sexual conduct which saw the clergy poking its nose into every aspect of its parishioners' sex lives.

First, there were the appropriate days for intercourse. Or, more accurately, the appropriate days on which to abstain. These included Thursdays (in memory of Christ's arrest); Fridays (in memory of his death); Saturdays (in honour of the Virgin Mary); Sundays (in honour of the Resurrection); Mondays (in commemoration of the departed), and every Tuesday or Wednesday in the three, five or seven days before communion as well as the forty days before Easter, Pentecost and Christmas.

Second, there were the appropriate positions for intercourse. Or, more accurately, the appropriate position, for there was only one: the missionary position. This, according to the medieval church's most august thinker, Thomas Aquinas, reflected man's superiority over women; to reverse or alter it (whether by having the woman on top or by engaging in sex *more canino* [in the fashion of dogs]) was to invite immediate ruin.

Third, there was the appropriate aim of intercourse, which meant only procreation. The further one deviated from this, the more heinous the act, with the curious result that homosexuality (in which two sets of semen were wasted) was a more serious offence than masturbation (in which only one set was wasted), which in turn was more serious than rape, incest, or adultery where semen (however unwelcome) might possibly be transformed into progeny.

Fourth, there was the appropriate mental attitude for intercourse, which, drawing on the teachings of Augustine, meant utterly without passion. And finally, there was the appropriate relationship for intercourse which, with a nod to St Paul, could only mean marriage. The Church had become increasingly involved in marriage from the fourth century onwards, but had resisted declaring it a sacrament, largely in deference to Jerome, until the twelfth century, when it became clear that they could profit more by controlling it than by railing against it. There were fees, therefore, for conducting weddings, blessing legitimate children, and investigating all manner of conjugal concerns, including, as we saw in the case of John of Canterbury, impotency.

It may seem, from the above injunctions, that the Christians of medieval times were trying to stamp out sex altogether, but in fact this was far from true. By the tenth century, the Church had established itself as the greatest power-base of medieval Europe, and it had to find a way to run the show. As an earthly power, it needed a people to prop it up, so some sort of compromise with the facts of life would have to be made. And just as it gained the formal power to tax people's incomes, so the Church decided to tax their souls, condemning acts which were wired irrevocably into their systems, and then selling them the means to salvation.

Thus began the extraordinary system of penitentials and confessionals, by which people were obliged to subjugate themselves to the rule of the Church by intoning Christian dogma, enduring ritualised punishments, or making cash donations every time they had a sinful thought. It was an idea as ingenious as it was devious, and it had people totting up their moral scores with the enthusiasm of football fans, never stopping to ask who invented the rules, whether they were absolute, or where their cash was going. In the same way that people became addicted to this sort of pay-as-you-go method of obtaining personal salvation, so the Church became addicted to collecting the proceeds, extending the repertoire of taxable offences as widely as possible and continually hiking the penalties.

But there was a problem. The obsessive detection, description and punishment of erotic offences began to feed straight back into the European libido. Even for the most devout and thoroughly committed Christian, determined to remain a virgin or to whittle their sexual life down to the bare minimum, the Church's own relentless emphasis on sex must have given rise to more sinful thoughts – and possibly actions – than would have arisen in a more relaxed regime. The preaching, allegories and images of Christian worship were starting to promote, in subtle ways, the very actions they decried, and even feeding the will to commit them.

Representations of Jesus began to take on a powerfully erotic tone – the agony of the early martyrs (especially St Sebastian) all too often appeared to be the ecstasy, and the Virgin Mary was slowly transmogrified from a symbol of sanctity into a sexual fetish, especially by the twelfth-century abbot of Clairvaux, St Bernard, and his followers, the Cistercians. And just as these figures became sexually charged, the devotion which they inspired became sexualised too. Among nuns, dreams of ecstatic union with Jesus became commonplace, and among priests, especially those given to punishing their own sinfulness with whips and cilices, religious devotion bled frequently into sexual fervour. The Acts of the Saints recounts many such tales, including that of St Felix of Cantalice, who, while conducting mass, would often become so transported with ecstasy that he was unable to speak, and that of Veronica Giuliani, who was so anxious to embrace the Lamb of God that she took a live lamb to bed with her, where she kissed it fervently and allowed it to suckle at her breast. Perhaps the most interesting example is St Teresa of Avila, who wrote of her communion with God himself in distinctly erotic terms, as follows:

An angel in bodily form, such as I am not in the habit of seeing except very rarely . . . not tall, but short, and very beautiful . . . In his hands I saw a great golden spear, and at the iron tip there appeared to be a point of fire. This he plunged into my heart several times so that it penetrated to my entrails. When he pulled it out, I felt that he took them with it, and left me utterly consumed with the great love of God. The pain was so severe that it made me utter several moans. The sweetness caused by this intense pain is so extreme that one cannot possibly wish it to cease, nor is one's soul content with anything but God . . .

Nor was this strange sexualisation of Christianity absent from the secular world. Church-instituted brothels flowered in much of Europe between the thirteenth and fifteenth centuries; randy monks, lusty nuns and prurient confessors became the stock-in-trade fantasy figures of prostitutes and pornographers; even in real life, the detailed and exhaustive lists of sexual sins read out by priests to their penitents may have been designed for the administration of punishment, but just as often functioned for the promotion of temptation. It went without saying that each unfortunate penitent was required to recite, in full, the details of his or her sin to the confessor. It is less well-known that sometimes part of the penance was to repeat the act with the confessor himself.

Sadomasochistic stirrings

Among all the sexual peculiarities engendered by medieval Christianity, perhaps the most interesting is that peculiar mingling of pleasure and pain, humiliation and triumph that we now categorise as sadomasochism. Outside the Christian West (and for different, though parallel, reasons, Japan), sadomasochism has never really taken off as a major sexual theme. Yet in Europe, as in the United States, sadomasochism in its broadest sense has become an integral part of our sexual subculture, accounting for a small but significant percentage of all professional sexual transactions and a considerably larger part of the imagery of commercial sex. Although there are hints of sadomasochistic tastes among the Romans, who recommended the bloodthirsty atmosphere of the arena as a fine place to conduct illicit affairs, and among the Indians, who were exhorted by the *Kama Sutra* to bite their partners, sadomasochism in its ritualised sexual form is proper to the Christian West. And it seems to have begun, like so much of our sexual heritage, with the priests and nuns of medieval times.

Perhaps the first stirrings occurred in the eleventh century, when the Franciscan monks began to extol self-flagellation as a penance. This practice was extended into the secular arena shortly afterwards, with priests stripping their errant parishioners naked and administering one hundred lashes in place of every previously intoned penitential psalm; a generous ratio, even then. Although it seemed cruel and mindless, the practice clearly had its rewards, for soon a number of particularly holy (and particularly sinful) people began to keep whips in their own homes and to flagellate themselves. The phenomenon grew steadily during the twelfth century, then suddenly exploded in the thirteenth, when thousands of self-declared flagellants began to organise themselves into processions and march through the medieval landscape, whipping themselves and each other as they went.

It was an extraordinary spectacle. The first outbreak occurred in northern Italy in 1259, where, as one historian wrote, 'day and night, long processions of all classes and ages, headed by priests carrying crosses and banners, perambulated the streets in double file, praying and flagellating themselves'. The local magistrates were appalled (not least because some of the flagellants were as young as five years old) and tried to expel them from their cities, but to no avail. The movement spread outwards to Germany, Austria, Bohemia, the Rhine province, the Netherlands, and even England, gathering converts as it went. Whole villages and even towns began downing tools to take up the whip, typically spending thirty-three and a half days scourging themselves, in memory of Christ's thirty-three and a half years of life. The alleged aim of the processions was to atone for the sins of the world and achieve grace in the hereafter, but the enthusiasm with which the flagellants whipped themselves, and the frenzied atmosphere in which the processions took place, point to more immediate rewards.

We now know that physical pain can produce an endorphin high similar to the thrill reported by skydivers or bungee-jumpers. We also know that concentrated bursts of anxiety excite sexual desire, a psychological process demonstrated in men by David Barlow, who threatened subjects with electric shocks only to find them getting uncharacteristically large erections, and in women by Donn Byrne, who recorded high arousal levels after his subjects had been embarrassingly obliged to perform public karaoke versions of the American national anthem.

These experiments help to account for the reward some people feel in dangerous or humiliating practices, but they are not sufficient to explain the whole phenomenon of sadomasochism. In S/M clubs today, there is a sense of theatre which equals, if not outweighs, the atmosphere of sexuality, an atmosphere which often draws heavily on Christian iconography and fetishes: the cross, the confessional, the miserable sinner and the unforgiving God. Certain themed S/M clubs in Europe and the United States contain rooms decked out like churches, with confession boxes in which clients can be humiliated and crosses on which they can be 'crucified'. Churches, of course, had no need to pretend, and we have an indication of the aphrodisiac power of medieval Christianity from the penances required of the clergy: a twenty-day fast for masturbation, rising to thirty days for masturbating in church.

Perhaps the clearest way to see how Christianity ploughed the furrow from which sadomasochism – this extreme yet archetypal expression of Western sexuality – would sprout is to compare the experiences of the priesthood with those of the self-proclaimed sadomasochist. Harry Walsh, a Catholic priest turned sexologist, remembers his days in the seminary, only a few decades ago, when he was obliged to wear barbed-wire bracelets with the hooks turned inwards, and to chastise himself with a knotted whip every time his thoughts turned to sex. Indeed, he recalls, 'Those who'd scourged themselves so hard they had blood on the walls of their cells were seen as occupying a higher rung on the spiritual ladder than the rest of us.'

In form, as well as content, this experience closely mirrors those of many S/M enthusiasts, one of whom was interviewed by sex researcher Martin Weinberg. When asked why he engaged in sadomasochistic practices, he replied, 'Because it is a healing process . . . the old wounds and unappeased hunger I nourish, I cleanse and I close the wound. I devise and mete out appropriate punishments for old, irrational sins . . . A good scene doesn't end with orgasm: it ends with catharsis.' Just as Harry Walsh wasn't talking, in his own case, about sex, this man hadn't been asked to talk about Christianity, yet in searching for an appropriate way to express his desires, he fell naturally and immediately into the script of sin, pain and redemption which drove the Christian Church and its followers for nearly two millennia.

From damnation to degeneracy

Cornflakes make a delicious breakfast cereal. Poured straight from the packet, doused with a generous helping of milk, and sprinkled with a little granulated sugar, they taste and feel as fresh as the fields from which their main ingredient was plucked, ground, baked, and dried. This image has not escaped the notice of advertisers. Successive television commercials, from the 1950s to the present day, have extolled the life-giving potential of the cornflake – its cleanliness, its wholesomeness, its energy – and above all, its family qualities.

Few would imagine that the clean-cut cornflake (and its cousins, Granola and the Graham Cracker) was at the epicentre of a dedicated attempt to shape Western sexuality which would be instrumental in revivifying Christian anti-sexualism just as its grip was beginning to loosen, and in shaping nineteenth- and twentieth-century sexual attitudes on both sides of the Atlantic.

The path began to be prepared after the English Reformation of 1534, then again as the pilgrims set sail for America. There were now two main factions to Christianity; on the one hand, the original Catholic Church, the genuine heir to Augustinian original sin and the whole package of guilt and redemption which went with it; and on the other, the rather more pragmatic, *laissez-faire* Protestants, who gave birth to the Puritans, who populated America from the seventeenth century onwards.

The attitudes of the Protestants and Puritans were rather different from those of the Catholics. They enjoyed a relatively rumbustious sexuality. Certainly, the Christian principles were there in the background, but they were tempered by realism, by the desire for converts, and by the need to populate the lands in which they had settled. As a result, the sexual *mores* to which they adhered bore a much closer relation to the ancient Jewish attitudes than to the medieval Christian ones, with a strong emphasis on procreation (to increase the numbers of the faithful), a hard line on adultery (to keep the peace), and a thunderous denunciation of all forms of non-procreative sex.

Things looked dangerously close to settling down into the sort of stern but pragmatic heterosexual orthodoxy which most burgeoning cultures have adopted in order to maximise growth. Close, that is, until yet another new lunatic fringe came to the fore, wedding ancient religious myths about sexual contamination with new-minted scientific myths about the causes and nature of disease. It was, literally, an unhealthy alliance, whose prejudice and dangers would not be equalled until the time of the Aids crisis two hundred years later.

The story starts with an anonymous tract called *Onania*, published in England in the early eighteenth century and attributed to a clergyman named Dr Bekkers. *Onania* concerned the practice of masturbation, and derived its name from the biblical figure of Onan, who had 'spilled his seed on the ground' rather than copulate with the wife of his deceased brother, as Jewish tradition demanded.

In one respect, *Onania* was typical of the attitudes of the times. It railed in the most colourful terms against the evils of masturbation and the sinfulness of those who indulged in it. But in another, it was revolutionary. Whereas all previous Western authorities had advised against masturbation from a moral and religious standpoint, *Onania* advised against it on medical grounds, suggesting that it was the prime cause of practically all the major disorders of the body, from ulcers and influenza, through childlessness and tuberculosis, to madness and even death.

To conjure up the process by which masturbation accounted for all these ills, Bekkers turned to the age-old theory of semen depletion, which held that semen was created, at great expense, from the blood, and that to waste it unnecessarily led to enfeeblement, anaemia, and susceptibility to disease. The Chinese had been using this idea to regulate the sexuality of their citizens for over two thousand years, but it had not been much in demand in the West, whose luminaries had preferred to threaten the everlasting souls of their people than the temporary bodies in which they dwelt.

However, a number of discoveries had recently been made which shook the age-old foundations of religious belief and which were beginning to suggest a new, more compelling, template for understanding both the world and our place within it – a template based not on religion but on science.

In 1632, Galileo Galilei had developed a sufficiently powerful telescope to observe in detail the canopy of the heavens, leading him to conclude that the Sun, and not the Earth, was at the centre of the Universe. Only a few decades later, his macroscopic feat was matched by the microscopic one of Anton van Leeuwenhoek, who developed a lens sufficiently powerful to investigate human semen, whereupon he noticed that it consisted not of a solid, dough-like substance from which babies were baked like buns in an oven, but of millions of tiny sperm, or *animalculae*, as he termed them, which performed the task of procreation.

With this new capacity to gaze in detail at the heavens which arched above us and at the world which dwelt within us, it became clear that science might have the wherewithal to challenge long-held religious dogma and to tackle convincingly some of the knotty questions of belief with which Christians, and people from all other faiths, had been wrestling for thousands of years. Where had we come from, where were we going, and what was our place in the Universe?

As a result, if the alarmist Dr Bekkers and others like him wished to convince people of the evils of sexual excess, masturbatory or otherwise, they were going to have to exchange the outmoded rhetoric of religious doctrine for the new lexicon of science. Since there was little apparent evidence to support Bekkers' case, he turned the clock back to ancient China, reinvented the myth of semen depletion, and dressed it up as a brand new scientific fact. This, then, is semen-depletion theory according to Dr Bekkers: 'The blood is made into Seed, which is further elaborated and purify'd in the Epidydimides . . . the oftner the Vesiculae Seminales are emptied, the more work is made for the Testicles, and consequently the Consumption of the finest and most Balsamick part of the blood.'

To the modern eye, it's complete quackery, but to the eighteenth-century readership, it was a new gospel. And, just like the traditional gospel, it came to be taught in schools, colleges and universities, eventually attracting disciples from all over the world.

In Europe, the chief advocate of semen-depletion theory was the Swiss physician Simon André Tissot, whose *Treatise on the Diseases Produced by Onanism* (1776) refashioned Bekkers' ideas under the label of *Degeneracy*, extended the list of diseases which could be caused by sexual excess, and now implicated women as well as men. Although women didn't possess any semen to deplete, they were weaker vessels, so the fluids they did excrete exerted just as damaging an effect. Tissot wrote, 'The symptoms which supervene in females, are explained like those in men. The secretion which they lose, being less valuable and less matured than the semen of the male, its loss does not enfeeble so promptly, but when they indulge in it to excess, as their nervous system is naturally weaker and more disposed to spasms, the symptoms are more violent.'

To back up this argument he called not on the effects of masturbation but on the grisly tale of a young prostitute who had allegedly had sex with six Spanish soldiers in a single night. She was brought the next morning into the southern French city of Montpellier, where she expired within hours, 'bathed in a uterine haemorrhage which flowed in a constant stream'. As with all Tissot's case studies, it was unsourced; even if true, it sounds more like the tale of a woman raped to death than one exhausted by her own lusts.

The book, with its doomsday tone and *faux*-scientific language, was a massive best-seller, making Tissot, as well as the doctors who benefited from his work, into the eighteenth-century equivalents of millionaires. Yet although none were averse to profiteering from the panic of an ill-informed populace, there may also have been another, rather more genuine basis for their concern.

From the early 1500s onwards, a number of particularly virulent strains of syphilis began to spread through the population of Europe, killing as many as one in twenty people at some points, and infecting as many as one in ten. At the time, there was no theory of how venereal diseases could spread; only the observation that they habitually affected those who were most sexually active. Furthermore, there was considerable confusion between the symptoms of syphilis, chancroid and gonorrhoea, which were often assumed to be a single disease. This, combined with the observation that those in mental asylums spent an unusual amount of time playing with their genitals, may have led Tissot and others like him to add two and two together only to make five, suggesting that frequent excitation of the genitals (whether through sexual union or the so-called 'solitary vice') was the culprit behind both physical and mental debility.

The snowball of degeneracy theory was now gathering speed at such a pace that it was not long before it crossed the Atlantic and arrived in America. Here, it would be adopted and preached, with an interesting new twist, by three of the most celebrated health reformers of the nineteenth century: Sylvester Graham, James Caleb Jackson and John Harvey Kellogg.

Rise and shine

In many ways, these three men were the scientific equivalents of Paul, Jerome and Augustine, sharing their combined enthusiasm for the thrills of public speaking and the horrors of sexual passion. However, whereas the Christian apologists blamed passion on the sin of disobedience, the new wave of nineteenth-century health reformers blamed it on a more distant and (to this day) more fashionable scapegoat: rich food and red meat. Accordingly, Graham, Jackson and Kellogg advocated a diet of strict vegetarianism, designed to dampen the sexual appetite and regulate the body in accordance with the pure principles of nature. But this was not all. For every passion that could be ingested through the mouth, Graham, Jackson and Kellogg believed that there were others which permeated the air and could be inhaled through the nose. These airborne passions were particularly fond of foul and polluted atmospheres, and preyed with special vigour on the sedentary. As a result, the three advocated special programmes of fresh air, exercise and cold showers – a regime of which Graham spoke in distinctly homoerotic tones and which Kellogg took so far as to squirt cold water up his rectum every morning.

Along with the dangers of rich food and the pollutions of foul air, the third cornerstone of these men's beliefs was that the passions thus raised could lead inexorably to debility and death. Although this idea was closely related to traditional degeneracy theory, it also represented a major advance, for whereas Tissot had pinned the cause of degeneracy on the loss of a physical substance, namely sperm or vaginal secretions, Graham, Jackson and Kellogg believed that passion itself was to blame. They were, in effect, Augustine to Tissot's Jerome.

After introducing the initial perils which befall those who engage in foul imaginings while masturbating, Graham described what happens if they persist:

> General mental decay continues with the continued abuses, till the wretched transgressor sinks into a miserable fatuity, and finally becomes a confirmed and degraded idiot, whose deeply sunken and vacant, glossy eye, and livid, shrivelled, ulcerous, toothless gums, and foetid breath, and feeble, broken voice, and emaciated and dwarfish and crooked body, and almost hairless head – covered, perhaps, with suppurating blisters and running sores – denote a premature old age! a blighted body – and a ruined soul!

To prevent their followers, and the American people in general, from turning into a race of disease-ridden zombies, dying off faster than they could be born, Graham, Jackson and Kellogg were convinced that there was only one cure. A long and (relatively) expensive sojourn at one of their resorts, during which the residents would be obliged to indulge in frequent exercise, eat their newly invented vegetarian breakfast cereals (the cornflake among them) and abstain, at all cost, from masturbation – the most unseemly summoning of passion and the most expensive waste of fluid.

Not only that, but Graham, Jackson and Kellogg also published a number of sexual advice books which the American people at large, especially those neither rich nor wise enough to visit their institutions or consume their cereals, could read, absorb and respond to.

These volumes all had a no-nonsense, practical, almost prim ring to them, yet their contents were the stuff of science fiction and their tone was almost rabid.

The thirty-nine signs

In one such book, *Plain Facts for Old and Young*, Kellogg indicates to parents how to spot masturbators among their children. It is made up of the so-called 'thirty-nine signs', so terrifying and all-encompassing that they damn, under one heading or another, every child in the land. Somewhat abridged from the initial descriptions he gave of them, the thirty-nine signs are as follows: general debility, consumption-like symptoms, premature and defective development, sudden changes in disposition, lassitude, sleeplessness, failure of mental capacity, fickleness, untrustworthiness, love of solitude, bashfulness, unnatural boldness, mock piety, being easily frightened, confusion of ideas, aversion to girls in boys but a decided liking for boys in girls, round shoulders, weak backs and stiffness of joints, paralysis of the lower extremities, unnatural gait, bad position in bed, lack of breast development in females, capricious appetite, fondness for unnatural and hurtful or irritating articles (such as salt, pepper, spices, vinegar, mustard, clay, slate pencils, plaster and chalk), disgust at simple food, use of tobacco, unnatural paleness, acne or pimples, biting of fingernails, shifty eyes, moist cold hands, palpitation of the heart, hysteria in females, chlorosis or greensickness, epileptic fits, bed-wetting, and the use of obscene words or phrases.

It was a list from which nobody was exempt, whatever their proclivities, yet just in case a child or teenager slipped under the net and escaped detection, Kellogg advised that it was probably not because they were innocent but simply because they were more canny, for 'the devotees of Moloch pursue their debasing practise with consummate cunning'. Therefore, parents were advised to keep a constant vigil on their children's sleeping habits, spying on them from outside their bedroom doors and listening for tell-tale sounds. 'If the suspected one becomes very quickly quiet after retiring,' he writes, 'the bedclothes should be quickly thrown off under some pretence. If, in the case of a boy, the penis is found in a state of erection, with the hands near the genitals, he may certainly be treated as a masturbator without any error . . . If the same course is pursued with girls . . . the clitoris will be found congested, with the other genital organs, which will also be moist from increased secretion.'

The 'remedies' to be meted out, in the new credo of John Harvey Kellogg, were perhaps the cruellest aspect of all his teachings. In the case of young boys, he recommended immediate circumcision without anaesthetic; in the case of young girls, the cure was even more extreme. What's more, it bore the imprimatur of a personal recommendation. He writes, 'in females, the author has found the application of pure carbolic acid to the clitoris an excellent means of allaying the abnormal excitement.'

Today, this sort of behaviour would qualify as child abuse, and Kellogg would be serving a lengthy prison sentence. But in those days he was the pompous judge, the ill-equipped jury and the sadistic prison-guard all in one, and he chose to incriminate the entire institution of childhood, for whom genital exploration, as we'll see in the next chapter, should have been a vital part of healthy sexual development. Had Kellogg's dictums been confined to the fringe, they might not have done so much harm. There have always been those, like the adherents to Heaven's Gate and disciples of the desert fathers, who seek refuge in extremes and find fulfilment in sadomasochism. But in Kellogg's case, the effect was far more widespread and the damage more enduring.

In Kellogg's lifetime, his books went through scores of reprints and were read by millions, from genteel Americans to farmers in the Australian outback. Far from being thought of as cranky or eccentric, they were sold by subscription book clubs and consulted by parents as reliable reference works of household medicine. What's more, his ideas filtered down, albeit in diluted form, into even the most orthodox texts, where they formed the backbone of mainstream thinking about sexuality for nearly a hundred years. In the late nineteenth century, a whole range of sadistic anti-masturbation contraptions were invented and marketed; in the early twentieth, young people who suffered from consumption were not taken to the doctor for fear that they would be branded masturbators; and as late as the Second World War, Scout manuals and sex-education films continued to warn children that masturbation was 'filthy' and that if they indulged, their bodies, as well as their minds, would suffer.

In a sense, the legacy of this thinking lingers on. For all their adherence to contemporary science, many professional football coaches still forbid their star players from having sex on the eve of important games for fear that it should sap their vital energies. Our inherited uneasiness about masturbation and 'irresponsible' sex has also hamstrung our response to a new sexual epidemic, Aids. As recently as 1994, when the US Surgeon-General Jocelyn Elders suggested, at a World Aids Day conference, that teenagers should be taught about masturbation as an integral part of

SHAPING FORCES

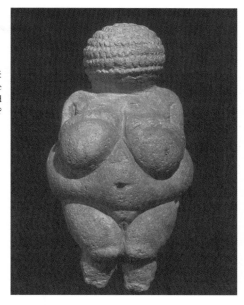

The Venus of Willendorf: matriarchal goddess, Stone Age centrefold or 30,000-year-old fertility symbol?

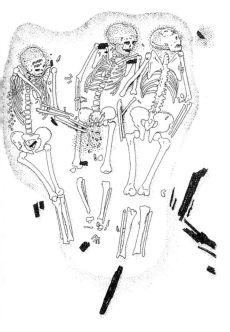

Sketch showing the 'Red Threesome', the Ice Age remains of two men and a woman found in a shallow grave in the Czech Republic. Is this the first formal record of humanity's violent sanctions against adultery?

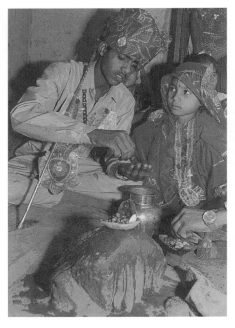

A five-year-old Indian bride watches her fifteen-year-old husband during their wedding ritual. In Rajasthan in August 1985, 50,000 children were promised to each other in a series of mass betrothals over two days.

Marriage, Western-style: a traditional British white wedding.

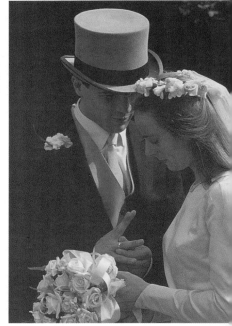

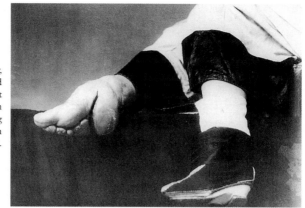

In the eleventh century, early Chinese women had their feet bound to prevent them from straying. Soon the results of the binding became a fetish in themselves.

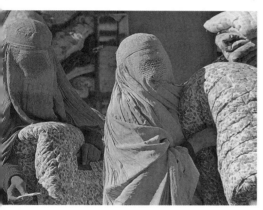

Afghan women living under the extreme Islamic code of the Taliban. Heavy veiling such as this sends a clear signal that these women are taken, and not available to any men other than their husbands.

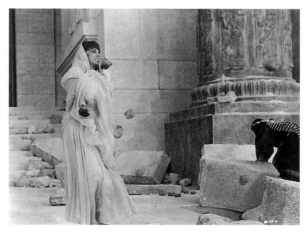

'The wages of sin is death.' Punishment by stoning, as portrayed by Gina Lollobrigida in King Vidor's *Solomon and Sheba*.

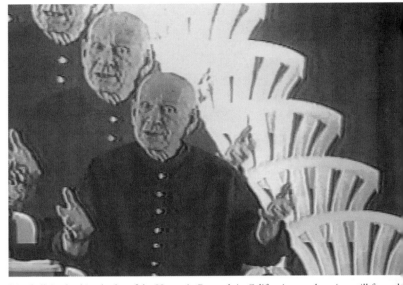

Marshall Applewhite, leader of the Heaven's Gate cult in California, seen here in a still from the videotape made shortly before he and thirty-eight others committed suicide.

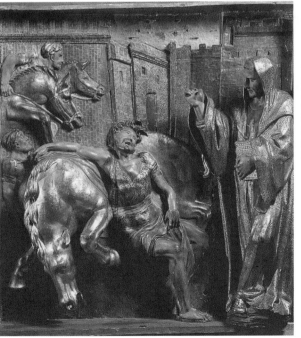

The Conversion of St Paul by Alonso Berruguete. Paul's famous letters to the Corinthians have formed the bedrock of Christian thinking on matters of sex and marriage ever since.

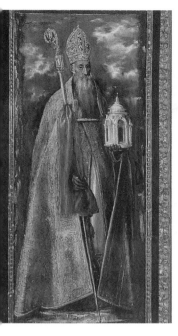

St Augustine by El Greco. According to Augustine, lust was not a natural part of creation but a disease introduced into human nature at the moment of the Fall, responsible for the expulsion from Eden and staining every generation from that day to this.

The Assumption of the Virgin by Titian. Following on from the teachings of Paul, Jerome and Augustine on the virtues of virginity, it became all the more essential to emphasise that Jesus himself had been born untainted by sin. His mother's virginity, therefore, soon grew from an apocryphal folk-tale to a central pillar of the Christian faith.

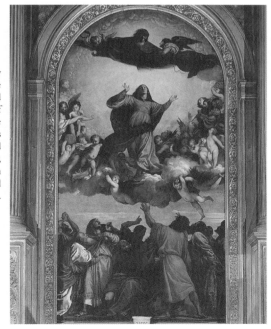

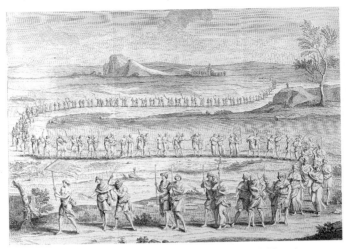

'Day and night, long processions of all classes and ages, headed by priests carrying crosses and banners, perambulated the streets in double file, praying and flagellating themselves.' By the mid-thirteenth century, self-flagellation had become a popular penance throughout Europe.

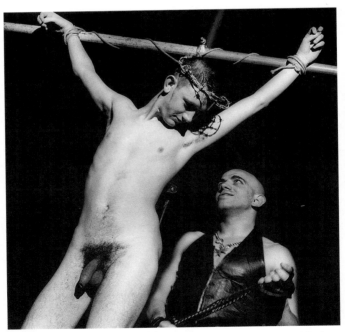

The S/M scene today often draws heavily on Christian iconography and fetishes: the cross, the confessional, the miserable sinner and the unforgiving God.

O N A N I A:

OR, THE

H E I N O U S   S I N

OF

𝕾𝖊𝖑𝖋~𝕻𝖔𝖑𝖑𝖚𝖙𝖎𝖔𝖓,

AND

All its Frightful Confequen-
ces, in both Sexes, Confidered

WITH

Spiritual and Phyſical ADVICE

to thoſe who have already injur'd themſelves
by this Abominable Practice.

To Which is Subjoin'd

A Letter from a Lady to the Author [very Curious]
concerning the Uſe and Abuſe of the Marriage-Bed with the Author's Anſwer.

*There shall in no wiſe enter into the Heavenly Jeruſalems
anything that defileth, or worketh Abomination. Rev. xxi.v.27*

𝕿𝖍𝖊 𝕱𝖔𝖚𝖗𝖙𝖍 𝕰𝖉𝖎𝖙𝖎𝖔𝖓

LONDON, Printed for the Author, and
at the *Bell* in the *Poultry*, *P. Varrenne* ;
Somerſet House in the *Strand*, and *J.*
Ball against *St. Dunstan's Church Flee*
Price 1s. stitch'd

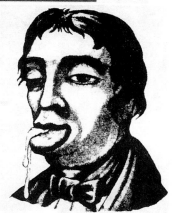

The book that started all the trouble: frontispiece
for an early edition of *Onania*, which railed in
the most colourful terms about the evils of
masturbation, with (right) one of the alleged
results, according to a Victorian health manual.

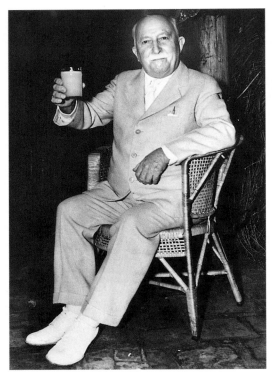

John Harvey Kellogg, cornflake-pioneer, prophet of degeneracy theory and author of the 'thirty-nine signs' shown by masturbators. His list was so comprehensive as to damn the entire populace at a stroke.

An advertisement for birth-con devices printed in Dr H. A. Allb *The Wife's Handbook*, first publ in 1886. It would be nearly an hundred years before contrace truly liberated women.

Condoms from the mid-nineteenth century, printed with erotic scenes.

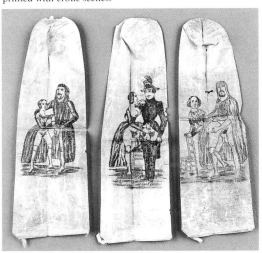

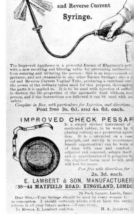

MALTHUSIAN APPLIANCES
The Improved Vertical
and Reverse Current
Syringe.

The Improved Appliance is a powerful Enema of Higginson's patt with a new receiving and filtering valve for preventing indisserted from entering and irritating the person; this is an improvement of pertance, and not obtainable in any other Enema Syringe; also a ent and Reverse Current Vaginal Tube, producing a continual curr the power of the ordinary tubes used for this purpose, thoroughly the parts it is applied to. It is to be used with injection of coffee to destroy the life properties of the spermatic fluid without inju person, and if the instructions are followed it can be used with ent safety.
Complete in Box, with particulars for Injection, and directions
Post free 3s. 6d. and 4s. 6d. each.

IMPROVED CHECK PESSAR
Is a simply devised instrument of
medicated rubber, to be worn by
playing coition] as a protection again
tion. It is c. astructed on a com
principle, and strictly in accordance
female organization; can be worn e
of time with ease and comfort,
adjusted and removed, adapts itself
and an apprehension of it going too f
the slightest harm need be felt, and
will last for years.
Post free with directions for
2s. 3d. each.

E. LAMBERT & SON, MANUFACTURER
138–44 MAYFIELD ROAD, KINGSLAND, LONDO

24 Park square, Leeds, June
Dear Sirs,—Your Syringe should be used by every woman t.
to conception. I should certainly advise you to have the verti
actions in all your future market.—Yours truly,
To Messrs. E. Lambert and Son.   H. A. ALLBUTT.

safe-sex education, there was instant outrage. That well-known moral champion, Bill Clinton, demanded and received her resignation the same day; but Elders still maintains she doesn't regret a single word.

Sexual revolutions

Under the weight of guilt and fear which Kellogg and others like him had inspired, some people at least continued to copulate, to masturbate and, presumably, to enjoy the experience. What they must have been waiting for was *proof*. Proof that Kellogg was wrong, that the Christians were wrong, that sex was neither inherently sinful nor the first step to physical ruin. Within a few short years they were to have it.

In 1861, the French chemist Louis Pasteur developed the concept of germ theory, which suggested that diseases were not caught through foul vapours or a surfeit of sexual activity but by the transmission of microbes in fluids. He was quickly proved right and, by 1905, the microbes responsible for gonorrhoea, soft chancre and syphilis had all been found. Fifty years later, thanks to the discovery of penicillin, they could also all be cured.

At the same time, huge leaps were being made in the technology of birth control. Until the mid-nineteenth century, most condoms had been handmade, and the process was laborious. One recipe says, 'Take the caecum of the sheep; soak it first in water, turn it on both sides, then repeat the operation in a weak lye solution of soda, which must be changed every four or five hours, for five or six successive times.' And this was before all the cleaning, cutting, shaping and stitching that would eventually ready them for use. The first real fuss over contraception followed in the wake of the development of vulcanised rubber in the 1840s, allowing barrier methods of birth control for women. After the emergence of crepe rubber a few decades later, and liquid latex in the 1920s, condoms could eventually be mass-produced and sold to an eager public via the newly invented vending machines which were placed in men's toilets, petrol stations, taverns and tobacconists.

Then, in 1960, came the Pill. Even though condoms and caps had been available for some time, it had never been easy for women to obtain them. The lingering legacy of anti-sexualism applied in particular to women, who (even when they were permitted to buy and use contraceptives), were made to feel uncomfortable at requesting them from chemists, ashamed at producing them from handbags, and awkward at being too familiar with their application. Diaphragms could be a little easier to live with, but many found them uncomfortable to fit and difficult to co-ordinate with the most propitious moments for intercourse. The Pill swept away all these difficulties. It was discreet, reliable, and it offered women the knowledge that they had round-the-clock, round-the-month protection, allowing them to engage in spontaneous bouts of passion without the need to stop, blush, and ask (or face) a barrage of awkward questions.

In large measure as a result of this new contraceptive technology, women were now beginning to enjoy an unprecedented degree of freedom. For more than ten millennia they had been under the authority of men, their fertility closely monitored and their activities curtailed and confined. All sorts of myths had been invented to sustain this situation. They were evil temptresses, who must be resisted; agents of chaos, who must be subdued; inferior beings, who should be ignored; weaker vessels, who deserved indulgence; or airy simpletons, who should be troubled by nothing but frippery.

By the 1960s, however, none of these myths held water any more. With much greater control over their own fertility, and the capacity to avoid pregnancy if they wished, women had much more say in their own lives. They could go to work and earn a professional wage; they could travel about with little or no male supervision; and they were notably less endangered by the consequences of their sexual activities. What's more, during this period, religious influence was probably at a lower ebb than at any other time in Western history.

This coming-together of female emancipation with the possibility of risk-free sex for both parties, all in an atmosphere of loosening religious restrictions, led to the shift in sexual attitudes and behaviour that we now term the Sexual Revolution. The consequences were slightly different for women than for men. Women did not immediately leap into bed with every man who passed. The evolutionary programme which had been planted in their brains over the four million years of human evolution was too deeply embedded to be cast away in a single generation.

Nevertheless, there were definite changes. At its most muted, the Sexual Revolution meant that couples were no longer stigmatised for having sex before they were married; that single people were free to engage in sex on a relatively casual basis; and that recreational sex, even in its oral, anal, or masturbatory varieties, was no longer automatically considered less valid or less healthy than the man-superior, peno-vaginal exercises in procreation which had held the moral high ground for more than five hundred years.

With an upturn in the number of orgasms per person per year, many traditionalists feared the worst. There would be moral decay among the young; a lack of respect for traditional values, which would threaten the fabric of society; a real danger of disease and destruction; even a new Sodom. But while many of the young did break away from the traditions that had held sway for the previous two thousand years, there were few signs that Armageddon was imminent. The flames of hell stayed well away, and venereal disease didn't wipe out the population at a stroke. Indeed, for a happy interval of around twenty years (before the advent of Aids), it seemed as though human sexuality had finally escaped the crippling double burden of unwanted pregnancy and lethal venereal disease which had suffocated it for millennia. Moreover, the vital strength of the Western world was not sapped or drained. In fact, there seemed to be a new energy, a new optimism. Anything seemed possible.

In some quarters, this optimism even led to the belief that, far from being the *source* of all misery, sex might even be the *cure* for all ills. The trend was started by magazines like *Health and Efficiency*, which eroticised fresh air and exercise by publishing photographs of sunkissed men and women enjoying cycle-rides and swimming jaunts in the nude, a move which no doubt had Kellogg turning in his grave.

Next were the sexual healers and therapists, who claimed to put people back 'in touch' with themselves through advocating (and often supplying) sensual massage, sexual exploration, and free and frequent orgasms. Although often open to abuse, many of these may have had a truly beneficial effect, combating the prevalence of vaginismus and impotence brought on by two millennia of fear, horror and mistrust.

Finally, at the furthest extreme of the new sexual gospel, were the free-love colonies like Kerista in San Francisco, Ganas on Staten Island, and Atlantis in Colombia. Here, wounded victims of sexual repression or self-styled sexual adventurers forged new lifestyles in which marriage, and all the ties which went with it, were thrown out of the window and sex between anybody and everybody was both encouraged and expected. Mildred Gordon, the fiery matriarch who still runs Ganas, a community of eighty such people on the east coast of America, remembers night after night of debate on how to refashion sexual relationships within less confined parameters: 'We had wondered for years why primary relationships had to be sexual and why sexual relationships had to be exclusive . . . If those things coincide, we thought, that's great, and if they don't – and they often didn't – why should we keep trying to make them do so?'

One can understand the sense of optimism with which such places started, bursting the bubble of so many centuries of anti-sexualism. Initially, it must have seemed extraordinarily liberating. A new Eden, without the Fall but with erections. A social and sexual nirvana in which few sexual favours were refused. Yet despite their best efforts and often serious intentions, the ultimate fate of most such communes was not so happy. And their denouement provides us with a fascinating final lesson about the shaping forces of history and culture, not just in the Christian West but throughout the world.

Free love takes a fall

In 1879, the man who invented the term 'free love', a pastor named John Humphrey Noyes, was obliged to flee his commune at Oneida in upstate New York after being accused of sexually initiating two teenage girls. In 1994, David Berg died in hiding amid accusations of sanctified prostitution and rampant child abuse within his cult, the Family of God. And in 1990s Oregon, the remaining shreds of the Rajneeshpuram commune, set up by the fraudulent Indian guru Bhagwan Sri Rajneesh, finally fell apart.

Although at first sight these seem exceptional and unrelated events, the result more of the weaknesses of their leaders than of any inherent tension within the group, the pattern in all was the same, and the deeper one looked, the more similar the stories became. At first, in many of the communes, total freedom had been the watchword: a return to nature, the absence of restrictions. But total freedom had not led to total happiness. Jealousies began to spring up, possessiveness took root, and consequent tensions developed between members. The tensions, in their turn, led to the adoption of rules, about who should sleep with whom, how often, and for what purpose. Habitually, the rules were fashioned by the leaders, and whatever their particulars, their direction was always the same. It was the leaders who decided the distribution of partners, and it was the leaders who usually ended up with the most. Noyes, for example, took it upon himself to sleep with the youngest, prettiest, most alluring women at Oneida for the greatest proportion of his time. More junior members, meanwhile, were palmed off with less frequent opportunities for congress and with much older partners. David Berg went further, requiring female cultists to go out on 'flirty fishing' expeditions – converting sceptical male outsiders by having sex with them – and demanding that even children should have sex indiscriminately. Everything, including sex, was to be shared without fear, and supposedly without favour; yet Berg, like other cult leaders, got the lion's share of sexual opportunities.

Sometimes the rules which the commune leaders devised were based on superstition, sometimes on personal bias, and sometimes on (usually ill-founded) scientific theories. Noyes, for instance, taught that there was an ascending fellowship of humanity more or less correlating with age, which dictated that the younger members of the community could receive the most spiritual benefit from sleeping with the older members, and vice versa. Being one of the oldest members himself, it was his burdensome duty to provide such opportunities for the young, just as it was their natural privilege to sleep with him. David Berg, Bhagwan Sri Rajneesh, David Koresh and many others all expounded similar views, and buttressed them with claims of divine authority. 'Everyone would have been happy to be David's wife if God so chose,' remembers one survivor of Waco. 'He used to say that God wanted some grandchildren.' The grandchildren were forthcoming: in addition to his own wife's children, Koresh fathered twelve others by six different women from the compound, many of whom were married to other men at the time.

Sooner or later, all this was bound to come to a head. With the commune leaders enjoying more than their fair share of partners, it was not long before some of their followers grew envious. And as we have already seen, sexually envious men become restless, and restless men eventually become violent, calling either for equal rights or an end to their leaders' excesses. In some circumstances, the leaders exert such control over the minds and hearts of their followers that they can defuse, at least temporarily, the situation. In others, they can keep them loyal to the end. This is what happened in Jonestown, for instance, and in Waco. But such absolute control usually requires the indoctrination of harsh, fascistic principles that cut against the logic of social living and can often end in disaster. In Waco, it led to the whole compound being burned to the ground; in Jonestown it led to mass suicide, and for followers of Rajneesh, to the community falling apart in a welter of acrimony and even cases of poisoning. In Oneida, Noyes had neither the power nor the will to resist the jealous outrage of his members. So during 1879, after the scandal with the two teenage girls, he fled to Canada. It was not long before the commune he had left behind imploded and collapsed.

Conclusion

However we try to get around it, or however false it feels, some form of sexual culture will always be with us, as profound and potent as the sexual nature upon which it is founded. It starts, often, as a genuine attempt to harness and control the potentially destructive side of human sexuality. Sometimes, it succeeds. But just as often, the myths and religions that are called on to justify its existence create a new sexual order, which favours the dominion of the powerful and which warps the sexuality of the credulous populace into strange new shapes. Under the strain, cultures must bend, adjust or break.

Christianity has fashioned a culture which advocates peace, selflessness and inclusion – at least for the converted and the virtuous. Yet in doing so, it has always felt the need to combat what it sees, not always erroneously, as the world's most selfish activity: sex. The fervour with which it has gone about this has led, through the ages, to guilt, obsession and a strict procreative orthodoxy which admits no variations and which is unmatched for its effect on both men and women by any other major culture. The regime seemed to have broken down in the 1960s, but today, in the wake of the failure of free-love experiments and the sudden advent of Aids, the old myths are being called on again, and their power seems as persuasive as ever.

Conservative politician Patrick J. Buchanan wrote in the *New York Post* in 1983 that Aids was nature's way of punishing homosexuals; James Anderton, the one-time Chief Constable of the Greater Manchester Police, attributed the spread of Aids to 'degenerate conduct' in the form of 'obnoxious sexual practices', and described gay men as 'swirling around in a cesspit of their own making'; and Lady Saltoun, a member of the House of Lords, warned recently that it was not possible for homosexuals to 'ge away from the wrath of God'. Even today, at the time of writing, the US Congress has just voted to spend $30 million per year on a campaign to teach children to say no to sex before marriage, on the alleged grounds that it is 'morally wrong'.

Christianity *per se* is not at fault. Its condemnation of sex has very often been balanced with an unusual stress on forgiveness and redemption, allowing it to carve a more constructive path towards human harmony than many of the world's other major religions. Yet for all their problems with misogyny, intolerance and violence, none of the other major religions has been as unstintingly, universally, and unequivocally negative about sex as Christianity, particularly Catholicism.

Today, in the wake of the failed free-love experiments of the 1960s and the Aids epidemic which is still with us, we should recognise more clearly than ever the need for controls on human sexuality, and for cultures which shape, direct and enforce them. But we must also recognise that all forms of human sexual expression, whether heterosexual or homosexual, procreative or recreative, can be as much a source of joy, happiness and human bonding as of jealousy, destruction and disease.

Recently, the Reverend Keith Walker of Winchester Cathedral suggested that the Christian faith is starting to move away from the idea of sex as original sin to the idea of sex as original blessing. Whether this will eventually be incorporated into the canon of new Christian thought remains to be seen, but it's an idea which leaves us with grounds for hope and, perhaps, for greater happiness.

PART THREE

THE SEXUAL SELF

The specifics of our individual sexual interests. How we acquire them and what they make us feel.

5

Different Strokes

On Sunday afternoons, about once a month, Gary Woolfe and his friend Peter load their car with two suitcases and set off up the M11 towards Epping Forest. Once there, they unload the cases and start laying out their equipment: bandages, a large holdall, two surgical tubes, a length of chain and a foot-pump. Gary gets undressed while Peter unzips the holdall and pulls out a large black body bag with a hard plastic carapace and a soft, inflatable interior. Wrapped from head to toe in the bandages, Gary then gets inside the bag, which Peter zips up around him. Peter inflates the bag with the foot-pump until it encloses Gary tightly, pokes two lengths of surgical tubing into his nostrils, then asks gently if he is all right. As soon as Gary hums a yes, Peter takes the chain, attaches one end to the bag, throws the other over the branch of a nearby tree, and starts pulling. When Gary has been hoisted about fifteen feet in the air, Peter secures the chain to the tree and walks away.

This form of solitary suspension is the only way in which Gary can become sexually aroused. He readily admits that it's not ideal, but conventional sex doesn't excite him. Women don't excite him. Men excite him a little, but he's too nervous to form relationships with them. And he won't go near rent-boys for fear of contracting HIV.

Gary's case presents a strange conundrum. It doesn't seem to fit in with any of the evolutionary strategies we identified in the first part of this book. Yet it's not culturally determined either. It isn't really about the Western cultural heritage of repression and guilt. What Gary finds arousing is the sensation of total enclosure, the feel of plastic pressing against his skin, the risk of being discovered and exposed, and the knowledge that it's Peter who's put him there.

It's a very specific and somewhat baroque sexual interest, and to ask how it arose is to identify the third major force which shapes human desire: the dictates of our individual constitution, both physical and mental. As well as being a sexually reproducing species, subject to the influences of our culture and history, every one also leads a highly individual life, with their own characteristic looks, their own defined personality, and their own family and friends.

It is these peculiarities of an individual's life which can narrow their sexual interest patterns down below the basic evolutionary drives, and beyond the influences of his or her culture, to the specific acts, scenarios and partners which they come to desire and, where possible, to enjoy. This third dimension of desire accounts for that part of our sexuality which we consider unique to us – our 'lovemap', as it is sometimes called – and it includes everything from our liking for boys or girls, blondes or brunettes; brains or brawn; people who do or don't look like our parents; breasts or buttocks; dominance or submission; and sex which is wild or tame. The sum of our individual sexual interests can be as personal, as varied, and as intricate as our fingerprints. So it's perhaps not surprising that the processes through which these interests develop is one of the most hotly debated areas in the whole of human sex research.

Born this way?

Alongside the sexual couplings demanded by evolution, varied sexual interests have always flourished too. History quickly tells us that human sexuality has never been limited to procreative acts alone. A taste for anal sex was widespread across many of the early civilisations; in Greece and Rome, homosexual paedophilia was institutionalised; and in Pharaonic Egypt there is some evidence that even necrophilia was not unknown. Herodotus states flatly that no male embalmer was permitted to be left alone with the corpse of a noble and beautiful woman for fear that he would ravish her. It's a fate, incidentally, which has befallen many of the world's most desirable women in more recent times, including, reportedly, Marilyn Monroe and Eva Perón.

But we humans aren't alone in our flexibility. It's worth noting that varied sexual interests, going far beyond the dictates of reproduction, exist in the animal world too. There are gay seagulls, masturbating porcupines (they use a stick) and lizards who seem to have pleasure and pain muddled up in a pretty sadomasochistic pattern.

A drive which extends no wider or deeper than to dictate straight-forward, orthodox coupling with an adult member of the opposite sex, is thus no more natural, normal or God-given than a lovemap which incorporates, for example, elements of bisexuality, or which ploughs more creative furrows away from the main highway of reproductive intent. Evolution would be a precision instrument indeed if it kept us so unswervingly on track as only to permit sex acts which included the possibility of procreation. Even if we accept that varied sexual interests are both normal and natural, we still have to explain how and why they exist. How do we acquire them? What purpose can they serve? In this respect, sexological opinion has traditionally been split into two sharply opposing camps.

On the one hand are those who feel that our sexual interests are all down to nature, that they are etched from birth into the architecture of our bodies and brains; innate, fixed, permanent. The ancient Greeks held this view about certain kinds of homosexual relations, arguing that men who preferred passive homosexuality had a misplaced organ of pleasure which could be reached only via the anus. Although this view of anatomy proved shaky, the idea that sexual orientation might be inborn has intrigued researchers from that day to this. Paradoxically, although we've moved ever further away from the Greek sexual regime in recent centuries, the idea that people are permanently and intrinsically gay or straight, and that these preferences are rooted in the body, has grown more powerful. These days, in deference to Darwin, explanations stressing nature tend to talk more about genes, or hormones, or brain structures, but the message is the same: sexual behaviour is the expression of inborn, unchangeable traits.

But there is another, equally powerful, lobby which suggests quite the reverse: that everything is down to nurture. According to this line of reasoning, we are born as a blank slate on which our culture, our family, our peer group, and our experiences in early life all conspire to shape our sexuality like sculptors with a lump of clay. In this schema, homosexuality (or indeed any other sexual interest pattern) is not innate; it is learned gradually and depends on who is influencing us when our sexual behaviour can be radically altered.

The debate between believers in nature and nurture is ancient, fiercely fought, and often fruitless. It's also riven with contradictions and shot through with ironies. For some decades in the West, the 'blank slate' view, claiming nurture is all, has been the property of tweedy sociologists, many on the left of the political spectrum. If we were blank slates, they argued sexual 'norms' could – even should – be challenged and sexual behaviour could change. Yet by the 1990s, some of the most vocal proponents of this view are the Christian New Rightists, who feel that since sexuality is acquired, they are legitimised in supporting attempts to try to change it. It's in the name of nurture, therefore, that electric shock treatment, aversion therapy and other strange and largely unsuccessful treatment have been prescribed for the 'cure' of homosexual desire.

Happily, however, the more we learn about the process of sexual development, the more it appears that neither camp has the monopoly on truth. Nature and nurture are not polar opposites, nor does one necessarily cancel out the influence of the other. In fact, nature and nurture are more like two sides of the same coin, with the former setting the initial template which the latter then refines and embellishes.

The reasons for this are subtle but important. If we lived in a totally predictable Universe, where neither the Earth nor any of its creatures changed, there would be no need for nurture at all: we could be completely pre-programmed and still prosper. Let's imagine, for example, that every man in the world looked like Tony Blair and every woman like Cherie. All we should need is a single genetic programme which told us to look out for partners with the appearance, smell, mannerisms and personality of the Blairs, and to desire whoever possessed them. But, as we know, life is not like that. We are a species subject to the laws of sexual reproduction, and sexual reproduction demands that every individual is different: some in subtle ways, and some in very dramatic ways. Moreover we're beset with other problems too: we have to balance the time and energy we spend on sex against our needs to find food and shelter, and to avoid getting ourselves killed.

In this unpredictable and constantly varying environment, the rigid hard-wiring of our sexual tastes would be disastrous. What if the particular set of qualities we were programmed to desire was absent from our vicinity, our species, or even our world? We'd have no chance at all of reproducing and our line would soon die out. There's simply no option. We have to be flexible, at least to some extent. This is why evolution has designed us to inherit only a bare minimum of innate rules for mate selection, leaving us to establish the rest only after we've been born and had a chance to assess the range of partners potentially available to us.

These rules, and their exceptions, begin, like so much that is fundamental to us, at the moment of conception.

'Thanks for the genes, Mom'

If genes which promote reproduction will multiply faster than others, then they should home in on situations where there's a reasonable chance of reproducing. So if there was one component to our sexuality that it would make most sense to inherit genetically, it would be an attraction to members of the opposite sex. At least some heterosexual leanings would seem to be a basic requirement for successful reproduction in any environment. Yet curiously, some of the strongest evidence that heterosexuality is hard-wired is the suggestion that homosexuality may be too, at least to some degree.

Michael Bailey, a psychologist at Northwestern University, Illinois, and Richard Pillard, a psychiatrist at Boston University, have made a number of studies into the genetic causes of sexual orientation by looking at the special case of identical twins. Because each identical twin shares almost exactly the same genetic material as his co-twin, Bailey and Pillard reckoned that if they could assemble enough pairs of identical twins and question them about their sexual orientation, they would have a reasonably good measure of whether genes were playing a role. In their most recent study, they managed to recruit fifty-six pairs of identical twins and fifty-four pairs of fraternal twins, by placing advertisements in gay publications asking gay men and women who had twin siblings, or adoptive siblings of the same sex, to come forward.

Their results were startling. About half of the identical twins had co-twins who were gay too. But in the case of the fraternal twins, who didn't share as many genes, only around 20 per cent of their co-twins were gay. And when Bailey and Pillard looked at adoptive siblings, the proportion of gay brothers and sisters dropped steeply, to only around one in ten. When they assessed these figures and compared them with the base-rate of homosexuality in the general population (which they took to be between 2 and 10 per cent), the researchers felt able to estimate that the genetic influence on sexual orientation must be between 30 and 70 per cent.

Bailey and Pillard's findings are intriguing, but they beg as many questions as they answer. If only half of the pairs of gay identical twins shared the same sexual orientation, then the other half, who still had the same genetic material, nevertheless had very different sexual tastes. If there really were genes for homosexuality, or even for heterosexuality for that matter, where were they, and what did they actually do?

The challenge was taken up by the ambitious geneticist Dean Hamer: bright-eyed, bushy-tailed, smooth-talking and sun-tanned. Hamer's lab is located in the prestigious National Institute of Health in Washington DC, where he has the kind of leeway most envied by scientists: to pursue his research interests with relative freedom. Although this perk is largely due to Hamer's groundbreaking work on the molecular genetics of cancer, he has now chosen to refocus his energies on to the thorniest areas of human sexuality.

Fuelled by Bailey and Pillard's work, Hamer spent two years at the NIH searching for the genetic basis for homosexuality, then announced in 1993 that he had found it. Overnight, he became a sensation. His claim was splashed across the front pages of newspapers, he was asked to appear on talk shows across the United States, and thousands of T-shirts with slogans like THANKS FOR THE GENES, MOM began to appear on the backs of gay activists from coast to coast.

What Hamer had done was to reconstruct the family trees of 114 gay male subjects, whom he'd recruited via adverts in the press, and then to analyse them for gay relations. His first finding was that these relations appeared to crop up twice as often on the mother's side as the father's. This was exactly the pattern he would expect if the gene was located on the X chromosome. A girl inherits two X chromosomes, one each from her father and mother; a boy inherits one X and one Y chromosome, and since the Y always comes from their father, the X must come from the mother. So Hamer had his first clue.

Hamer's next step was to assemble forty pairs of gay brothers and examine their DNA. Upon doing so, he discovered that more than 75 per cent shared exactly the same configuration of markers in one particular region of their X chromosome, a region known as Xq28. It seemed impossible that this statistic had been arrived at by chance alone. If there really was a gay gene, here was where it must lie.

At this point, Hamer's research began to be questioned. First, Xq28 was not a single gene, as the media had assumed, but a large number of genes working within, genetically speaking, an extremely wide territory. Among other things, it was the location where markers for colour-blindness, haemophilia and some forms of diabetes had also been found. And second, if this gene really did make men gay, how could it have been transmitted through the generations? If one assumed that gay men would on average have bred less often than straight men, surely the ruthless winnowing-out of natural selection would have filtered it out long ago.

Hamer demurred to the first question. He had never claimed it was a single gene, he said, but he had proved there was a genetic basis and pinpointed the area in which the gene, or complement of genes, might lie. It was the newspapers who were responsible for the head-lines.

To the second question, his answer was more developed. Borrowing the logic of the eminent evolutionary biologist Robert Trivers, Hamer suggested that the so-called gay gene might not code for homosexuality as such, and certainly not for exclusively homosexual behaviour. Perhaps it might code instead for sexual attraction to males. If so, its presence in females would be highly advantageous, making them especially likely to seek out sex and reproduce. In males, however, its expression might point to a malfunction during foetal development in which a natural switch for suppressing it had somehow failed. If that were the case, it would only be a small minority of men for whom it would act as a gay gene. For those men in whom it had been 'switched off', and for all women, it would more closely resemble a straight gene.

As yet, Hamer's findings, and his theories arising from them, must remain speculative. They have still not been replicated by other research-ers and there is still no clear measure of the degree of influence genes might exert. Meanwhile, as scientists argue over the validity of his findings and sexual politicians over its implications, Hamer himself has moved on. He has mounted more questionnaires and family studies, investigating the possibility that there is a genetic component to the frequency with which individuals want to have sex, and that this genetic influence can be pinpointed to the serotonin transporter gene. Even more controversially, he has ventured into exploring whether the number of partners with whom we wish to have sex is also genetically determined, varying with the length of our dopamine D4 receptor genes.

The row over genes has perhaps produced more heat than light. And lest we forget, sexual behaviour might originate in our genes, but it has to be expressed through our bodies. What then are the other sources of our developing sexuality?

From genes to hormones

After a new individual has been conceived, its first four or five weeks of development are, sexually speaking, relatively uneventful. Although we tend to think that human beings come in two kinds, male and female, and that they have been that way since conception, the reality is actually a little more complicated. It's perfectly true that the genetic sex of each individual is set the moment they are conceived, yet this is actually only the first stage in a process of sexual differentiation that lasts for much of the time the child is in the womb.

What happens is this. For the first four or five weeks after conception, each individual develops along a predetermined line which varies little whether it is male or female. It has a dual set of tiny undeveloped tubes, which will become either the sperm ducts or the fallopian tubes, and a little clump of ambiguous cells which will become either the scrotum and penis or the vagina and clitoris. Should this state of affairs continue into the sixth or seventh week, with no input from any hormonal substances, the foetus will develop along female lines and be born as a little girl. However, should the foetus be flooded with testosterone (which with boys should happen naturally at around this time at a signal from the Y chromosome), the genitals, body and brain will divert themselves from the typical female path and follow the male one instead. The scrotal sac differentiates from the proto-labia, the penis emerges out of what otherwise would have become a clitoris, and the brain is rewired to respond to a diet of testosterone and related male hormones rather than oestrogen and related female ones.

It's one of the most finely tuned processes we're programmed to undergo. Yet in common with all natural processes, it's open to deflection and to error, for major irregularities in the amount of testosterone released during this period can have startling effects on the developing individual, blurring the lines between male and female. Crossing them over. Mixing them up. Should a male foetus not produce enough testosterone, or should its body be incapable of using it, the baby will be born with the internal reproductive organs of a boy but the external genitals of a girl. On the other hand, should a female foetus produce too much testosterone, as in a rare condition known as congenital adrenal hyperplasia (CAH), the child will have the internal reproductive organs of a girl but external genitals which more closely resemble those of a boy.

One of the major treatment centres for hormonal disorders of this kind is the Johns Hopkins University School of Medicine in Baltimore, where Ray Tyles, a CAH patient now in his late forties, is still undergoing treatment. Despite the fact that Ray was born with what looked like a small penis, the doctors who delivered him told his parents that he was a little girl, and he was taken home as 'Constance'. It wasn't until his first nappy change that they noticed the irregularity and rang the hospital in shock. After numerous examinations, Ray was diagnosed as having CAH, and it was decided that he might do better as a little boy after all. At the age of six, he began a traumatic series of operations: his genitals were surgically enhanced so that they looked unequivocally masculine, and he was renamed Ray.

With such a potent effect on the body of a developing foetus, it's not unreasonable to suppose that a surplus or a deficiency of testosterone might affect the mind as well. And, according to the latest research, this seems to be the case. Ray remembers that despite living his earliest years as a girl, he was never comfortable in the role. He wanted to act like a boy, he wanted to play like a boy, he felt like a boy. Now, he is convinced that even if he'd gone without the surgery and remained more like a girl physically, he would have grown up to adopt the attraction patterns of a boy.

In one aspect Ray was lucky. His doctor was John Money, possibly the most eminent sexologist in the world, and a man as insistent on his patients' rights to be themselves as he is dismissive of simplistic views of sexual identity and behaviour. Money agrees that Ray's feelings were not all that unusual. In a study conducted in the early 1980s, he found that even among CAH patients brought up as women, about 50 per cent had unusually masculine personalities and were unusually masculine in their behaviour. Furthermore, almost exactly the same number turned out to be attracted either partially or exclusively to women, a far higher proportion than in the female population as a whole.

Money's work suggests that the levels of hormones circulating in our bloodstream in the critical months before birth may be crucial in helping to sculpt not only the sex of our bodies, but the sex of our minds as well. Hormones usually help to create a masculine gender identity and a masculine sexual orientation pattern for males, and feminine gender identity and feminine sexual orientation for females; a kind of sexual road-map which, from then on, remains largely fixed. Given the complexity of our genetic inheritance, our hormonal balance and the human societies we grow up in, however, things may not always go so smoothly. Money points out that what we consider the basic pattern of sexuality actually rests on three different conditions: the sex we physically are; the sex we emotionally feel ourselves to be; and the sex of the people we desire.

For much of Money's career, the idea that sexual orientation or identity might be rooted in our bodies was out of favour. Investigating brains or hormones felt uncomfortably close to body fascism. Upbringing, not nature, was all the rage at the time. But today, as we delve ever further into hormones and the working of the body and the brain, with ever more sophisticated mind-mapping technology, it's becoming increasingly clear that Money, and those who agreed with him, were right. It's even becoming clear where some of these orientation centres might lie.

The sexual brain

In 1991, Simon LeVay published the results of a study in which he had examined the brains of a number of gay and straight men who had died of Aids, a number of straight men who had died of other causes, and those of a number of women. When he had analysed the structures of these brains 'blind' – that is, not knowing which brain belonged to whom – LeVay had found that a certain cluster of nuclei within the medial preoptic area of the hypothalamus (known as INAH-3) was smaller in the brains of the gay men than the straight men, whatever the cause of death. It had been known for some time that the medial preoptic area was implicated in sexual behaviour, and also that it was habitually larger in men than in women. What LeVay's finding seemed to suggest was that gay men had female-style hypothalami; in other words, hypothalami which did not differentiate under the influence of testosterone. In LeVay's subjects, it was not clear whether the testosterone had failed to reach the brain in sufficient quantities, or whether the men simply didn't have a mechanism for accepting all that was destined to hit them. What was clear, however, was that this could be the first tangible proof that gay men might have a physically different mindset from straight men, and that this mindset might have nothing to do with their upbringing, and everything to do with their birth. As LeVay dryly put it in his book *The Sexual Brain*, 'perhaps gay men just don't have the brain cells to be attracted to women'.

Seven years on, and LeVay's experiment is still the subject of fierce debate. Aids wreaks havoc in the brain, sometimes causing severe dementia and blindness, so the brains may not have been typical of healthy humans, whether gay or straight. Also, it's possible that the difference in the size of INAH-3 might have been a *result* of the men's homosexuality, not its cause. But as time goes on and an increasing number of similar experiments come to light, LeVay's basic claim – that gay people and straight people have different brains and that these differences may help to account for deep-rooted and ineradicable differences in their sexuality – seems to become more and more credible.

Of the more recent studies, perhaps the two most interesting have been conducted by Laura Allen and Roger Gorski at the University of California at Los Angeles, and by Dick Swaab, at the Institute of Brain Research in Amsterdam. Allen and Gorski focused their study on the anterior commissure of the corpus callosum (the connective matter which joins the left-hand side of the brain to the right-hand side). They found, rather like LeVay, that the anterior commissures of gay men much more closely resembled those of women than those of other men. Swaab, on the other hand, completed in 1995 an examination of six male-to-female transsexuals and found a size difference that appeared to correlate neither with sex nor with sexual orientation but only with sexual identity; that is, the sex which the transsexuals emotionally felt themselves to be. Although at first sight perplexing, this finding is particularly significant since it suggests that there might be at least two separate components involved in our underlying sexuality (orientation on the one hand and identity on the other), each differentiating under the influence of prenatal hormones and each with its own neural locus.

It might be that both of these areas are affected by the same surplus or lack of testosterone, explaining why some gay men seem effeminate and some lesbian women butch. Yet it is just as possible for testosterone to affect only one of the crucial areas, leaving the other untouched. This might help to explain why just as many gay people also appear to be 'straight-acting', different from their straight counterparts only in the sex of the person they desire. The same can hold true in mirror image, with some exclusively straight men exhibiting a leaning towards femininity, and some women seeming atypically butch while still being attracted only to men.

Again, these findings are highly controversial, and as yet they remain unreplicated. The mind-boggling complexity of the human body makes it dangerous to draw conclusions too easily. Nevertheless, there is growing conviction across most branches of the sexological community that this complement of three prenatal factors (genes, hormones and brain organisation) together set the stage for the most fundamental aspects of sexuality. Not only the sex we are, the sex we feel, and the sex we desire, but maybe even the strength of our sex drive, and possibly the degree to which we seek sexual variety. What is less certain is the degree to which they do so. In his more cautious moods, even Dean Hamer warns against the over-interpretation of his data, suggesting that the gay gene may be responsible for only a small percentage of our orientation. And let's remember those pairs of identical twins in the Bailey–Pillard studies, where one twin was gay and the other straight, despite the fact that their genes were virtually identical and that their hormonal environment in the womb must have been markedly similar. There must be other, postnatal, factors at work which serve to reinforce, complement, or over-ride our basic biological predispositions, and which start to turn the barest outlines of our sexuality into a much more complex, much more fully rounded picture.

These other factors begin to take root from the moment we leave the womb.

From the womb to the world

For babies who reach full term, birth must be a rude awakening. After nine months in the safe, predictable environment of the womb, we are suddenly exposed to a whole new world. Our eyes are open, our fingers explore. Sight, touch, smell, hearing, taste. Our five senses alert us to a massive range of possible experiences, some of which will settle and become arousing while others inspire immediate and permanent aversion. But how do we pick our way through this minefield of virgin sensations? How do we understand the possibilities and assess the range?

Cindy Hazan has some clues. For many years, she has been studying the process by which infants become attached to their parents and the consequences when the process doesn't go well. From the moment they leave the womb, babies will reach out helplessly, gaze at the person in front of them, and cry for attention. Hazan and her colleagues believe that they are starting to exercise one of the most potent weapons in the whole armoury of human survival techniques: the attachment mechanism.

In the 1940s, a team of pioneering researchers, including child psychologists John Bowlby, Mary Ainsworth, and James and Joyce Robertson, undertook a project in which they filmed scores of babies and young children, watching for their reactions when they were separated from, or reunited with, their parents. At the time, children's wards in hospitals were institutional, regimented places, where parents were discouraged from visiting lest they upset the children. Not that the staff were unkind: the babies in their care were fed, sheltered, and kept warm. Yet the babies, without exception, were terribly distressed. First, they would protest, screaming, crying and searching for their mothers. More upsetting yet, if their calls weren't answered, they would slump into passive despair. After this stage, even if the parents returned, they would greet any further human contact either with raging anger, anxious clinging, or total detachment.

The babies were clearly and definitely expecting human interaction with care-giving adults, and when they didn't get it, even if they were fed and warm and able to survive, they were deeply upset. Furthermore, when they did interact with adults, they displayed a range of behaviours which, deliberate or not, functioned to keep those adults interested and attentive. Babies would gaze at their carers, reach out for them, cling to them, mirror their expressions and engage in gurgling 'conversations' with them. The Robertsons, and a whole generation of relationship psychologists in their wake, have used these films and the techniques they illustrate to argue that attachment is a universal process, with its roots in the evolutionary imperative to survive. They conjecture that children are born with an inbuilt range of behaviours which draw their parents towards them, where they can effectively be mesmerised, allowing a bond of attachment to take root which will ensure that the baby develops safely and securely. Attachment isn't just the foundation for later psychological development: it's a baby's best chance for survival.

Most parents follow the baby's lead and abandon themselves to care-giving with an enthusiasm born from unconditional love – hard-wired love. In these circumstances, the baby's early development progresses along predictable lines. As a newborn, although it can distinguish its mother by smell, its bids for attention can be satisfied by a wide range of people. But as a baby grows older, it becomes more attached to specific people, especially the 'primary care-giver', most often the mother. From the age of seven months or so, as the infant begins to crawl, it can be satisfied by few people except its primary care-givers, and strangers are treated with caution, even alarm. Attachment behaviour – demanding, clingy, and often very loud – comes to a peak as the child reaches toddler age and relies on its care-givers as a safe home-base during wider explorations of the world. But as long as the child can feel confident that its needs are likely to be met, and that the world is a largely benign and predictable place, such explicit demands ebb away and the young boy or girl develops more and more independence. This is the ideal programme, and it happens with around 60 per cent of all children, who become well-adjusted and securely attached to their care-givers.

Unfortunately, some parents are unable to provide the unconditional love and continued attention that their child demands. Some may be absent for long periods of time, others may simply fail to bond; yet others might be going through personal disturbances (health crises, domestic violence, family disruption) which prevent the formation of healthy, stable relationships of any kind. In these cases, the infant may develop along quite different lines, acquiring disorders of attachment that profoundly affect the way it relates to other people. If its care-givers are unpredictable, sometimes responding and sometimes not, the child may become so confused it will be more than usually clingy, so desperate for attention that it will never leave their side – a pattern Mary Ainsworth christened 'anxious/ambivalent'. If the care-givers consistently ignore the child's bids for comfort, the picture is still worse: the child will withdraw into itself, ignoring them, no longer seeking contact and retreating into a pattern termed 'avoidant'. More recently, it's been recognised that if the care-givers' reactions are so unpredictable (due to abuse, depression or disturbance) that the child has no idea what response it will get, it will itself behave in a completely disorganised way, sometimes clinging to and sometimes avoiding them. Finally, and most tragically of all, studies by Bowlby and his successors found that those infants in orphanages and institutions who had no opportunity to form any attachments at all often developed physical illnesses, suffered greater rates of depression and suicide, and found it extremely difficult to bond with anyone in later life.

Hazan and her colleagues, who have considered these disorders at length, believe that they are vital in helping us to understand the mechanisms at work in normative childhood development. But more than that, they also believe they can tell us something about the much later process of sexual attraction.

By watching adult lovers, courting and meeting in public places, Hazan and her fellow investigators were able to identify a predictable set of sequential behaviours which followed exactly the pattern of parent/infant attachment they had identified earlier. When they met for their first date, a couple who were attracted to each other would engage in the same complex dance, with an initial demand for attention (here a friendly chat-up line rather than an ear-piercing squall), typically followed over the course of an evening by light touching, shy smiling, increasingly confident mutual gazes and, finally, the close mirroring of each other's gestures; the sweeping of hair from the face, the timing of sips from a wine glass, even the sharing of food.

Furthermore, relationships begun in this way seemed to progress over time in much the same pattern as early attachment, moving from a period of pre-attachment, in which the object sought was relatively unfamiliar and the response could be provided by a variety of partners, to an exclusive romantic interest in one person, to the deep attachment of two lovers, to the well-adjusted partnership of a long-term marriage, where it was back to life as usual.

Just as the adult attraction scenario seemed to resemble the parent/infant attachment process, employing the same mechanisms in roughly the same sequence, so Hazan and her colleagues speculated that adult relationships might bring with them some of the legacy of actual childhood experiences. To find out more, she and fellow psychologist Phillip Shaver placed a questionnaire about love and attachment in one of Denver, Colorado's largest newspapers, the *Rocky Mountain News*. Over six hundred replies were analysed, along with over a hundred responses from 'captive' university students. All those questioned were given descriptions of secure, anxious and avoidant attachment, and asked to identify themselves as being of one type or another. They were then asked further questions about their experience of love as adults.

Those who had developed avoidant patterns of attachment, most likely as a result of being repeatedly ignored or rejected, admitted they were most likely to want to keep their partners at a distance. They hated emotional highs and lows and went to some lengths to avoid great involvement; they were less jealous, but also less concerned about intimacy. The anxious/ambivalent lovers, by contrast, who'd possibly been fazed by their parents' inconsistent reactions, were precisely the opposite: intense, needy and attention-seeking. They were highly jealous and more likely to be obsessive; they also believed more in love at first sight and the power of love, and felt sexual attraction and the need for reciprocation more keenly. By contrast, the majority of people, who identified themselves as 'secure', not only gave more positive accounts of love and sex, but had relationships which lasted for longer: they tended to endure for around ten years, compared to 5.97 years for the 'avoidants' and a stressful 4.98 years for the anxious/ambivalents.

The link between infant attachment and adult attraction finds further, anecdotal support in the observation that baby-talk is an integral part of many romantic partnerships, and also in the suggestion that many people come to desire those who look, act, or smell like their parents. In one study, conducted by Glenn Wilson, people were found to select romantic partners with the same eye colour as their opposite sex parent; in another, conducted by the American psychologist Art Aron, a large preponderance of newly-wed men and women were both found to have chosen spouses who closely resembled their mothers.

But although the work of John Bowlby, the Robertsons and Hazan is compelling, and may help to explain many of our long-held intuitions about the effects of parenting on later sexual relationships, many people come to desire individuals and scenarios which have very little in common with either their parents or the relationship they had with them.

Other, more complex forces must also be at work.

Neural networks

Gene Abel, at the Behavioral Medicine Institute of Atlanta, has specialised in the wilder shores of sexual interest for more than a quarter of a century, and is often called upon to account for sexual behaviour patterns which are so unusual or extreme that they have landed their practitioners in court. Abel's frizz of white hair, his distracted manner, and wildly gesticulating hands can make him look like a kindly caricature of a nutty professor; yet he nevertheless possesses one of the sharpest minds in the sexological community today.

From his personal experience of hundreds of cases, Abel has come to believe that we learn our sexual interests early; that we learn them by associating our own experiences with pleasant or unpleasant sensations; that we learn them gradually; and that once we have learned them, they cannot be easily unlearned. He cites for the purposes of illustration the story of a man who arrived in his office with six hours of videotapes, each of which contained nothing but shots of women's hands. On the fourth finger of each hand, a wedding ring was prominently displayed, and in some of the shots, the rings were being twirled or caressed.

The man had acquired these videos by approaching women in the streets of his home town and telling them that he planned to get married but had been unable to find a suitable wedding ring for his sweetheart, until he had happened to see theirs. Could he possibly film it with his video camera to help him find a similar one himself? The women, usually flattered, complied with his request, whereupon the man ran home, slotted the footage into his video player, and began masturbating. Unfortunately, the whole thing came to a head a few years later when he really did decide to get married. His wife loved him deeply but found it difficult to accept that he couldn't achieve orgasm unless he was staring intently at her wedding ring, and usually playing with it as well. If she took it off, or if it was out of sight, he was entirely impotent.

In trying to explain how his client might have developed such a bizarre pattern of arousal, Abel had to go beyond prenatal influence or parenting styles. Plainly, however unusual a mix of hormones his client might have been bathed in, they couldn't have brought forth such a specific and unusual problem. Abel's analysis of his client's condition had to look at his later childhood, and how he might have come to be so fixated on such a mysterious stimulus. To do so, he would have to tap into a new school of thought on brain development.

When we are born, our brains might already be hard-wired with the basic rules for astounding feats of manipulation, attachment and language, but in some ways they're also amazingly unformed and flexible. There's scope for almost any new experience to mould the very structure of our brains, to make new connections between cells and form physical pathways to help us survive.

Yet as soon as we start to develop, imbibing the smells, colours and shapes of the world in which we find ourselves, our connective matter, and the cells which lie between them, change too. Distinct pathways are formed which relate to certain oft-felt sensations and oft-repeated experiences. Others, which are unused, fall away. Gradually, during our formative years, the cells and pathways in our brain reorganise themselves, taking less diffuse, more delineated shapes. Networks develop in which our experiences, and our emotional reactions to those experiences, are etched invisibly yet ineradicably.

The period of the most frenetic development of these pathways is the first eighteen months of life, with the result that this is a vital period for our developing sexuality. Should we come to associate succour at our mother's nipple with comfort and reward, then comfort and reward may be sparked by physical closeness and warmth later in life. Should we be rejected, smothered or maltreated, then rejection, smothering or maltreatment may take root instead.

All this new brain activity means that something has to give. Those pathways which aren't often used will die away, the better to delineate and cement the rest, the better to economise. Nevertheless, plenty of virgin pathways remain, and new connections are formed relatively easily through to the age of about eight. Here, with most of the essential pathways established and the plainly useless or one-offs forgotten, the brain begins to slow down. Paths are less easily forged, memories and experiences less enduringly or effectively stored. This is not to say that new experiences can't be introduced and new associations made. Like taking up a new language or a musical instrument, it's perfectly possible to start at any age. It's just that the older one gets, the more difficult it is to progress from rote learning to the sort of instinctive, easy recall that signals virgin storage space and swiftly made connections.

By the age of around thirteen or fourteen, the brain has completed most of its major clear-outs, consolidating the useful pathways and junking the superfluous ones. The brain is now as developed in fundamental structure as it ever will be; individual, complete, fully formed. What is stored within it is the programme for life, the tastes, experiences, and skills that will endure.

As a result of new research into these processes, pioneered by John Holland and Gerald Edelman and still very much in its infancy, sexologists are now beginning to understand that the earlier a child is presented with a stimulus, the more impact it can have on the internal architecture of its brain. But it's not just the punctuality of the stimulus which is crucial. It has to be repeated as well. Repetition, in fact, was one of the most important factors in understanding why Gene Abel's client was fixated on women's wedding rings.

Abel explains the story by referring back to the man's early childhood, during which he received regular visits from an aunt whom he found particularly beautiful. His aunt would periodically encourage him to sit on her lap, where he became mesmerised by her habit of twirling a wedding ring on her fourth finger. She often took the ring off, and handed it to him to play with: an activity which he came to associate with his aunt, and through his attraction for his aunt, with his own sensory pleasure. From that time on, he was hooked, locked in a sort of feedback loop which made sure this particular attraction pattern grew ever more fixed in his imagination and, literally, in his brain.

Yet despite the fact that this individual's fetish resulted from the repetition of a pleasurable activity, the association doesn't always have to be pleasant, nor the later activity benign. According to Abel, and to most of the sexological community, powerful infantile stimulation of any kind is likely to set patterns of high arousal which may endure permanently. This might help to explain the fact that, although physical abuse, sexual abuse, and mental humiliation are profoundly traumatic experiences, a disproportionately high number of children who were abused become abusers in their adult life. As they engage in their sadistic behaviour, abusers come to identify with both the aggressor and the victim. As the aggressor, they avenge their own childhood humiliations. And as the victim, they repeat the activities deeply associated with the pattern of their own life: painful but comforting in their familiarity.

Much of the stimulation which children receive is from their parents. Typically, it is their parents who chide and admonish them and their parents who provide them with rewards. Yet the more such influences are examined, the more it becomes clear that it is not just the parents who guide the child's developing sexuality, nudging it gradually down one channel or another. It is also the child's peers, and in particular the way those peers interact with them.

Thus, having been born with a predisposition to desire either men or women, having established the style of relationship we will enjoy from our parents, and having picked up some of our own particularities of taste from the stimulation of our early years, we have already acquired the major aspects of our personal sexual template. And we're only five years old. Now, we're about to begin experimenting. And our experimentation typically takes two principal forms: sex play and gender play.

Sex play and gender play

School, it is often said, is a rehearsal for adult life. We learn how to make friends, how to forge alliances, and how to deal with the various complex tasks that will face us when we grow up. But as well as learning our social and academic skills at school, new research is showing that we also learn our sexual skills there. And this learning process, though less formal, is no less crucial.

Thore Langfeldt is a Norwegian sexologist who has pioneered research into the sexual development of children. By studying them at play, Langfeldt noted that if they felt they were unobserved, children from the age of four or five would often clasp each other and engage in rhythmic rocking movements which simulated sexual intercourse. They weren't orgasmic, or at least not usually, but they were certainly practising the same sorts of manoeuvres and feeling the same sorts of pleasurable sensations which adults experience during sex later in life.

In cultures where such behaviour is not frowned upon, almost all children engage in sex play and it seems to be a part of regular, healthy development. John Money, whom we met at the beginning of this chapter, attributes the near-universal sexual health of the Aborigines of Arnhem Land, with whom he's lived and among whom he's acknowledged as a traditional elder, to the fact that childhood sex play is fully endorsed. Furthermore, he notes, even among our primate cousins, individuals who are separated from their playmates and unable to engage in clasping and mounting behaviours develop into impotent and neurotic adults.

Left unsupervised, many children are fully aware of the sexual content of their games. Sometimes these involve masturbation, which, typically, begins by the age of fifteen or sixteen months, and sometimes mutual genital exploration. At least half of all boys, it's now thought, have had some sort of sex play with other children by the age of ten, while for girls, the figure is about one-third.

Occasionally children even engage in full face-to-face intercourse.

Theresa Crenshaw, a sex therapist from San Diego who also hosts a radio show called 'Love Soup', recounts a story in which a married couple were debating whether or not to let their two young children, Eric and Erin, watch an impending rape scene on their television. Before they had fully decided, the scene began, whereupon Eric turned to his parents and asked, 'Mommie, what's that man doing to that woman?' 'He's putting his penis into her,' replied his mother, 'but he's not doing it right. He shouldn't do it unless they both want to and he should make sure they love each other first.' 'Oh,' piped up Eric, 'well, I've tried to put my penis in Erin several times but it's too small and it keeps falling out.' The parents rang Crenshaw in shock, asking what they should do. Crenshaw replied that the children's feelings were perfectly natural but that actual intercourse would be better left until they had grown up and met other people whom they loved, when Eric's penis would also stand a greater chance of fitting.

In our culture, of course, where sex has until recently been a dirty word and children considered the last bastion of innocence, most signs of juvenile sexual interest have been vigorously suppressed. Yet even where this is still the case, children continue to indulge in sublimated or socially acceptable alternatives like 'Mummies and Daddies' or 'Doctors and Nurses', where kissing, cuddling and genital inspection can be presented to adults as carefree and blameless experimentation.

Sex play is an important part of our overall sexual learning process, teaching us how to provide sexual pleasure and how to respond to it. But it's not the whole story. Equally important is another aspect of our day-to-day childhood experimentation: gender play. Psychologist Melissa Hines has spent a lot of time examining the process by which we come to be male or female, masculine or feminine, straight or gay. And much of her research has been conducted in the classroom – or the playroom.

In one study, Hines set a number of toys down in a playgroup for two- to four-year-olds and observed which children played with which toys. Almost straight away, the boys gravitated to the trucks and the girls to the dolls. This didn't surprise her; nor did it prove anything about the origin of such preferences. What did interest her was that when she introduced the same toys to girls who had been exposed to unusually high levels of prenatal testosterone, they almost universally went for the trucks. Perhaps there was indeed something about prenatal brain organisation which pushed boys down a typically masculine path of development and girls down a typically feminine one.

But how much of this behaviour was inborn and how much was being learned as the children grew up? To test this, psychiatrist Richard Green assembled mixed-sex groups of children and asked them to perform a number of tasks, including telling a story and throwing a ball. Aware that there is a typical male way to throw a ball and a typical female way, dictated more by the physique of the two sexes rather than any stylistic preference, he was looking for exceptions. Quickly enough, he identified a small number of boys who threw in the female style, more from the wrist than the shoulder. There was nothing unusual about them physically, but psychologically, the majority showed some sort of gender discordance. They felt themselves to be 'sissy' and were often labelled 'sissy' by their classmates.

What seemed to have happened was that these particular boys had felt from a very young age that they didn't quite fit in, that they were not typical of their sex. This may have been down to prenatal hormonal imbalances or to altered brain structures. Alternatively, it may have occurred extremely early in their lives, as a result of their relationship with their parents. Whatever the reason, these boys, unable to identify with others of their own sex, had started to identify with the girls instead, copying their play patterns, adopting their interests, and even imitating their physical mannerisms.

Furthermore, as Green followed the development of boys such as these through puberty and into adult life, he found that 80 per cent turned out be sexually oriented towards other men. Not only had they adopted more of the characteristics and mannerisms of the opposite sex, they shared their sexual attraction to men.

It's difficult to ascertain whether boys who feel out of place with the rigid stereotypes of their gender voluntarily feminise themselves, or whether they are forced to do so as a result of being ostracised by their same-sex peers. What is certain is that whatever the biological substrate to gender development, some aspect of learning is involved as well. That aspect appears to be picked up partly from the classroom, and is largely in place before the age of eight.

From peer groups to paraphilias

In the case of normal, healthy children, the ideal prescription is to allow them to engage in sex play without permitting it to become an over-riding concern, and to allow them to adopt the gender identity consistent with their sex without being too disconcerted by departures from traditional ideals of masculinity and femininity. In this task, parents are usually aided by the child itself and, as a result, children have the chance to experiment with friends, learn from their peers, and be guided by their parents towards a sexual interest pattern that is socially accepted, easily managed and often rewarding. Many children can also get by without strong parental guidance, and some, without explicit guidance of any sort.

However, despite the remarkable resilience of young children, there are two parental responses which are almost guaranteed to set them off along more unusual paths. One is the radical over-collaboration with sex and gender play, and the other is the complete banishment of any kind of sexual behaviour. Pushing a child too early into sexual experiences, especially at the hands of adults rather than peers, can have a traumatic and devastating effect, as in the case of victims of sexual abuse. Similarly, forbidding the child from obtaining any knowledge or experience of sex as he or she reaches puberty can be equally damaging. Among those who acquire the most extreme form of sexual obsessions, known as paraphilias (including rape, bestiality and necrophilia), more than half report being brought up in households where any talk about sex was savagely forbidden. Nelson Cooper, who became obsessed with self-asphyxiation and whose autobiography *Breathless Orgasm* was published in 1991, recalls how he knew so little about sex that the first time he had a wet dream, he thought he'd found a way of expressing human milk. Similarly, Karen Greenlee, who as an adult came to desire only corpses, states that she remembers being fascinated by dead bodies from the age of five or six, when she watched John F. Kennedy's funeral procession on television, but felt at such a remove from her parents that she was unable to discuss her feelings with them, and unable to have her predilection halted.

Without the confidence to experiment with sex, and without the capacity to talk about it with their parents, Nelson and others like him become much more vulnerable to having their learning veer off in unusual and often inconvenient directions. When the whole issue of sexuality seems so disgusting and dangerous, John Money argues, even the most bizarre paraphilia can develop as a way of diverting one's sexual feelings into channels where there is less risk of rejection, revulsion or punishment. Paraphilias can, in fact, be seen as a workable way of coping.

Mark Matthews, who has written a memoir called *The Horseman*, and who runs an Internet site for those like himself who desire only animals, recalls that the best thing about the pony with whom he lost his virginity was that 'she couldn't laugh at me'. As a boy, Mark was repeatedly counselled on the evils of sex by his parents. Then, when he was caught one day engaging in sex play with his cousin, his mother thrashed him. 'She told me that I was evil,' he writes, 'that I was dirty, that touching girls was a terrible sin and would make me grow up to be a crazy man who would be locked up in the crazy house . . . and that I should never try to do that to a girl ever 'again in my life.' A few years later, when he reached his early teens, his burgeoning sex drive and profound fear of women combined to make him seek his first sexual experience in a farmyard by placing his hand inside a mare's vagina. Over the next two or three years, he masturbated to images of naked women, but with the memory of the mare at the back of his mind. Then, at the age of sixteen, lonely, overweight, and very low in self-esteem, he asked a classmate to accompany him to the school prom. She rejected him outright, describing him as a 'sick, greasy-grind brainhead who would be fit only for a pig'. 'At that moment,' Mark recalls, 'I gave up hope of any girl in that school, that town, that country, maybe the world, wanting to have anything to do with me.' He went to a nearby field and, desperate for some release, happened upon a young mare with whom he engaged in full intercourse. He would never look back, and now lives with some sense of well-being on a trailer park in the American Midwest with his equine 'wife', Dottie.

Trapped in gender

Just as the over-zealous promotion or fierce forbidding of childhood sexuality can radically redirect an individual's developing sexual interest pattern, the same is true of the way we treat gender. Too rigid or too enforced a collaboration with prescriptive ideals, with ridicule or punishment for non-conformism, and the child can come to wear its gender like a tight-fitting shoe, removing the mould only at night, in private, or when the pressure becomes untenable. Nelson Cooper, as well as being interested in asphyxiating himself, possessed strong transvestite yearnings. He remembers dressing up in his sister's flower-girl costume and telling his mother he wished he could go into a machine and come out the other end as a girl. He was laughed to scorn by his mother, and his desires went underground, expressing themselves later in his habit of masturbating while wearing only a tiny pair of bikini briefs.

It's an interesting quirk of sexual psychology that over 90 per cent of those identified by psychologists as having paraphilias are male. Some argue that the rewiring of the brain by testosterone in the womb, laying the template for male sexual desire over a basically female physical blueprint, might be the source of later confusion. But the same processes of repression or abuse which can lead to paraphilias in men can produce similar disruption to sexual behaviour in women.

Indeed, for girls, the subscription to gender ideals can be even more damaging. Many households still subscribe to rigid and stereotypical views about gender, with boys being taught that their domain is power, adventure and responsibility and girls that they are by nature submissive and should strive towards contentment, passivity and care-giving. Any behaviour which seems to threaten these categories is ridiculed, derided and abused; and as girls have traditionally been more restricted than boys, gender stereotypes fall particularly heavily on them. When gender ideals are too rigorously enforced, girls can come to suffer from profound resentment, which expresses itself in later revenge activities directed at their parents, their culture and their gender. Under this rubric, psychoanalysts have started to classify a whole new range of problems as specifically female perversions, which differ in interesting ways from the paraphilias usually found in men. While male paraphilias tend to be oriented to objects outside the body, and to be aimed specifically at sexual climax, female disorders tend to affect the whole body, or can emerge as patterns of apparently non-sexual behaviour. Among these patterns are shoplifting, anorexia and self-mutilation.

It's sometimes difficult, in the shifting sands of sexual norms, to draw the line between experimental sexual behaviour and full-blown paraphilia. Yet the latter, characterised less by a passing interest and more by an exclusive and obsessive yearning for unusual partners or activities, are very rare – affecting less than 1 per cent of the population. Moreover, they are often the result not just of misparenting or unhappy schooldays, but of learning difficulties and sometimes brain anomalies as well. Ron Langevin in Toronto has conducted studies which suggest that more than 40 per cent of sadistic sexual offenders have anomalies in the left-hand side of the brain, while Stephen Hucker, now at Queen's University, Ontario, has shown that similar numbers of paedophiles are affected in the right-hand side. Similarly, Fred Berlin, at the National Institute for Sexual Trauma in Baltimore, has found that paraphiliacs possess a vastly disproportionate number of various unusual physical conditions, from chromosomal disorders through hormonal imbalances, to brain anomalies of many different kinds. Physical conditions like these don't lead inevitably to paraphilias, nor do they lie behind every case of paraphilic desire, but there's no doubt that, along with parental abuse and unhappy experiences with one's peers, they can play a significant role.

The net result

By the time we reach puberty, all the forces designed to act upon us and almost all the stages we have been designed to undergo are complete. Genes, hormones, prenatal brain organisation, parent/infant attachment, one-off imprinting, neural network development, sex play, gender play, and peer-group learning. Sometimes, all these forces agree, nudging us without conflict down the path of exclusively heterosexual, completely gender concordant, perfectly furrowed sexual desire with no dents or deviations, no frills or fancies. Straight as a die. This, however, is the exception rather than the rule.

Most people, even if they categorise themselves as perfectly mainstream, will have picked up their own little set of idiosyncrasies. Once we venture into the world of fantasies, through the extensive letters collected by Nancy Friday and others, or between the covers of mass-market pornographic magazines, there are always twists and twirls, elaborations on the basic theme. Minor elements of bondage or submission; indications of same-sex leanings; and, in the magazines, pages and pages of advertisements for phone-lines narrating tales of urination, domination, spanking and submission. These publications are designed to connect with the greatest number of people in the shortest possible time, and while, like advertising, they can certainly influence some people's choices (if only by letting them know about things they might otherwise not know exist), they simply would not survive if the market showed no intrinsic interest. Commercial sexual material might be able to spark off crazes for one sexual activity or another, but they can't introduce entirely new varieties of human desire. They're not perverting an otherwise upstanding readership: they are catering to the deeply entrenched sexual interests of Mr and Mrs Average.

Mainstream pornography is now the largest media business in the world, topping both the movie and the music industries. In 1996, more than $8 billion was spent on it in the United States alone. But those with more specialist pornographic interests also exist in sufficient numbers to make minority publications a lucrative concern. Among the best-known are *Skin Two* and *Shiny International* for fetishists; *Hog Tied* and *Maitresse* for bondage and discipline fans; *Fifty Plus* for those with a special interest in post-menopausal women; *Paedika* and *Lollitots* for those who desire peripubescent boys or girls; and *Juggs* for those whose sexual interests include pregnant and lactating mothers. There are even highly specialised desktop-produced magazines like *Azrael* for necrophiles and *Squish* for those who have a predilection for being stamped on like tiny, worthless insects.

Human interest, as I hope I have shown, is exceptionally pliable, winding its way to fruition through a complex system of interlocking forces designed to make it flex in response to the vagaries of each person's individual circumstances. Yet underneath the flexibility we all show, with everyone having slightly different sexual tastes and many having radically varying ones, evolution has ensured that there remain several safety nets which function to keep the vast majority of us toeing the main line of reproductive potential – whatever our additional interests. Some of these, as we have seen, involve trying to hard-wire us for heterosexuality; some involve presenting us with our parents at key stages in our early develop-ment; some even involve our friends and classmates. But underneath these clear and usually helpful cues, there is still a further layer; a layer which kicks in with a vengeance when we reach the next and final major stage in sexual development – puberty.

Puberty

Sometimes it crashes through our dreams like a train in the night, sometimes it creeps up slowly, taking us by stealth and changing us gently, by degrees. Desire – no longer the soft-edged yearning of our earlier years, but the full-on, gut-wrenching, giddy-making experience of hot-blooded lust, heart-pumping arousal, and fully-fledged genital orgasm.

With many teenagers, the first purposeful masturbatory session heralds not only their entry into sexual maturity, but also the first full realisation of their truest, rawest desires. For most, this will involve an image or story centring around a sexually mature partner of the opposite sex. But for some, it may not. Those with less sanctioned sexual interests often don't discover their true desires until later. One of Dean Hamer's gay geners didn't recognise his homosexuality until after he got married, and divorced, when he decided to answer an advert for people seeking bisexual experiences and found he preferred the feel and smell of a man to that of a woman. Despite the fact that he'd had very few same-sex experiences before, it suddenly felt like the most natural thing in the world.

Although her tastes were very different, Karen Greenlee experienced similar problems. She'd been aroused and interested by death ever since childhood, but felt so remote from her strict parents that any discussion of her fascination was completely impossible. Time after time, she had tried unsuccessfully to date both boys and girls before she found herself alone one afternoon with a young, naked corpse. As an apprentice embalmer, she'd grown accustomed to dealing with the dead, but that one afternoon even Karen was taken aback by the force of her desires. She recalls: 'I'd been embalming and I was moving about. I got water or something on the floor, and my foot slipped. I fell down and my lips touched this guy's arm. I fell on top of him, and that was it. It was like lightning bolts, claps of thunder. It was like . . . I'm home.'

Discovering the best expression of one's sexual interests, and progressing from fantasy to real sexual activity, isn't easy for anyone. Even for those whose desires are pretty mainstream, it can be a trial to find a willing and available partner. Paraphiliacs have an altogether more difficult time: they might find their sexual interests constrained by the law as well as by their own lack of self-awareness. For some of us, in our most desperate teenage hours, it might have seemed a better idea to give up altogether. But for those who don't quite get it right first time, the massive surge of sex hormones that triggers puberty (testosterone for boys, oestrogen for girls), ensures that they feel sufficiently aroused sufficiently frequently to carry on experimenting until they hit the button. Often, this involves trying out a wide variety of masturbatory fantasies and a wide variety of experiences, some of them homosexual, some heterosexual, some perhaps incestuous, some even bestial.

The psychological changes that characterise puberty aren't the whole story, of course. There are dramatic physical changes too. In the case of boys, the back broadens, the frame lengthens, hair grows over many parts of the body, and the whole face begins to take on a lupine, muzzle-like quality with protruding cheekbones tapering to a long, straight nose and a large lower jaw. In the case of girls, sexual development follows a different path. Here, the face develops chiefly in its upper sphere, with fat pads enhancing the protuberance of the cheekbones and the eyes glistening and growing further apart. The body changes are different too. Breasts develop and the hips widen, so that the overall figure takes on the characteristic hourglass shape of a fertile woman.

It is these physical changes, to the frame, the face, and the curvature of the body, which make up the final safety net on the main road towards reproduction. This net consists of a whole range of adaptations which encourage us to pick out and respond to partners of either sex who display signs of maximal fertility. Curiously, it is these adaptations for recognising and responding to fertility out of which our whole perception of beauty is formed. For whether we are straight or gay fertility, at root, is what beauty is all about.

Universal beauty

When he was four years old, David Marquardt's mother was involved in a car crash. She flew head-first through the windscreen, breaking several bones and shredding her face completely. Doctors rushed her to hospital and performed a series of emergency operations before the young David was allowed to visit her. When he did, he was shocked. Instead of the smiling, soothing face which usually greeted him, he remembers that 'she looked like a monster'. Her teeth were wired together, her jaw was broken, her nose was crushed, and stitches perforated her entire face. David ran from the hospital screaming.

Several weeks later, his mother returned home. David had been promised she would be back to her old self, but she wasn't. She looked like a different person. Literally. Different eyes, different nose, different cheekbones, different chin. What's more, she acted differently too. David remembers, 'It was weird. Everyone told me she was my mother, but she was like a completely new person. She even talked differently.'

As he grew up, the image of his mother in the hospital and his reaction to her rebuilt face haunted David. He became obsessed by beauty, dating a string of beautiful women and training first as a dentist, then as a plastic surgeon. Slowly, he began to feel that there was something strangely similar about all the beautiful people he was seeing – and working on. Something nearly mathematical, almost architectural. It made him uneasy, and since he knew that the idea of a universal beauty wasn't exactly popular, he kept it to himself. Nevertheless, in his private life, David was busy. He studied the history of ideas about beauty, from the Greeks through to the Pre-Raphaelites, and found that despite the vast differences between the writers, in terms of period and culture, many had come to remarkably similar conclusions.

The most intriguing theory, in David's mind, was one of the earliest. According to Plato, all beautiful things conformed to a golden mean, which could be expressed as a ratio of approximately $1 : 1.5$. In terms of the human face, this meant that the distance from the hairline to the mouth should be 1.5 times the distance from the mouth to the chin, that the distance from the eyes to the chin should be 1.5 times the distance from the hairline to the eyes, and that the distance from the hairline to the chin should be 1.5 times the distance from one ear to the other. In more recent times, it had also been suggested that the golden mean might also apply to particular facial features, with the ideal mouth being 1.5 times as wide as the nose, and the ideal teeth being 1.5 times as high as they were wide.

Marquardt became fascinated by the golden mean, and wondered whether he could use it as a standard to judge every feature of every face, and all the relationships between them. He assembled a large collection of portraits and started work, drawing geometrical shapes all over them and scrutinising the results. At first, his efforts were in vain. However hard he tried, certain features eluded the ideal. Then he had a breakthrough. By envisaging the ratio as a series of pentagons rather than a series of rectangles with straight lines, he could map the face in much more detail. What's more, the faces began to fit.

Soon, he believed he had cracked the code. There was indeed an ideal ratio, it was very close to what Plato had predicted, and it applied to all the features of the face and all the connections between them. The ratio was 1 : 1.618 and it could be drawn, as a sort of mask, and laid over any face. The closer the face fitted, the more beautiful Marquardt found it.

To see whether this was a quirk of his own individual taste or a more widespread phenomenon, Marquardt invited a number of people up to his office and asked them to arrange a series of twenty faces in order of attractiveness. Everyone arranged the faces in exactly the same order, and in every case, the higher the rating, the closer the fit. In an exercise to try to find the world's most perfect fit, Marquardt then started laying his mask over portraits of models and movie stars. Among today's names, Cindy Crawford and Whitney Houston come closest. Among yesterday's, the 1970s model Karen Graham and the young Marlon Brando.

Marquardt's methods may seem a little home-made, and his data is certainly skewed in favour of Western looks, but the idea that we all have the same underlying notion of beauty, and that it conforms to certain geometrical standards, is finding ever-growing support among those who have been studying human beauty – not out of personal obsession or for professional gain, but in the more rarefied world of academia.

According to Donald Symons at the University of California at Santa Barbara, there are a number of features that people from all cultures and all walks of life reliably find beautiful, not simply because they are culturally idealised, but because they tap into our deepest reproductive urges and conform to a template which signals maximum reproductive potential: youth, fecundity, health, disease resistance and genetic quality. According to Symons, our brains are attuned to pick out and respond to such cues, converting them into the sensations of pleasure and delight that characterise our reaction to beauty. The total sum of such cues, in Symons's view, represents the various facets of beauty, and though they may be overlaid, refined or amended according to fashion, cultural variation, or personal taste, they remain stable and constant underneath.

The first and most obvious cue to health, and therefore beauty, is the envelope in which we all come wrapped, our skin. Across nearly all cultures, and in practically every part of the world, women whose skin is slightly lighter than the ethnic average have traditionally been considered more alluring than those whose skin is darker. In Japan, well before contact with the West, women painted their faces with chalk to make them appear more beautiful; in India, pharmacists have long plied a lucrative trade in skin-whitening products like Fair and Lovely and My Fair Lady, while in Europe (before Coco Chanel started sunbathing on the French Riviera and started a craze for tans), a fair skin was, sometimes literally, to die for. On one famous occasion in the seventeenth century, a Signora Toffana introduced such a powerful skin bleach into the Italian court that six hundred men were poisoned to death simply from kissing their wives.

Pierre van den Berghe and Peter Frost, who have studied perceptions of attractiveness in relation to skin colour, attribute the near-universal preference for pallor to the fact that our skin lightens at puberty, then darkens again with age and, in the case of women, with each successive pregnancy. As a result, the lighter-skinned women of any race tend to be its more nubile women, currently fertile but unencumbered with children and with all their reproductive years in front of them. In the modern world, where we deal with complex, multi-ethnic societies and a legacy of many unhappy interactions between races, preference for one skin colour or another is a lot more complicated. Yet in ancestral times, when we would have known a relatively small circle of pretty similar people, we'd simply never have encountered major differences in skin colour – for example, the differences between people of different races – so our fertility radar could home in on skin lightness with ease.

Skin is not the only thing that becomes darker as we age. Among Westerners, our hair does too. Whatever its underlying colour, it starts relatively light, darkens gradually through childhood, brightens at puberty, then slowly fades to grey. At the moment of maximum lightness, women are again at their peak of nubility. Blondes may have more fun, to elaborate on a popular phrase, because they look as if they can have more babies. Yet blondes are outdone, in one respect, by brunettes and redheads, whose darker, more striking hair can set off a fine pale face and better display the other dimensions of follicular attractiveness, body and shine. In either sex, a full head of luxuriant hair is a powerful indicator of youth, health, and therefore beauty. No shampoo has been advertised for its promise to turn hair grey, lank, thin or greasy.

The colour and texture of our skin and hair would have been potent signals of reproductive potential, especially in ancestral times. Yet people's bodies are equally rich in clues, and one of the most important of these, especially in the case of a woman, concerns the size of her waist in relation to the size of her hips.

'36–24–36'

At first sight, this seems like a rather random dimension on which to base judgements of attractiveness. Surely, waist-to-hip ratios are so varied and so subject to fashion that no meaningful generalisations can be made. The Venus of Willendorf, with her grossly exaggerated hips, bears very little relation to the graceful, classically proportioned Venus de Milo, who in her turn has little in common with the more voluptuous, Rubenesque quality of Botticelli's Venus. What's more, none of them bears the slightest relation to waif-like supermodels such as Kate Moss and Jodie Kidd. Yet Devendra Singh, an ingenious psychologist at the University of Texas, begs to differ. Singh, who has made the waist-to-hip ratio his life's work, began investigating body shape to discover whether there were any constant themes underneath the cultural and historical variations. If people were able to make judgements of attractiveness based one each other's shape, what exactly were they looking for?

He began by studying the changing dimensions of *Playboy* centrefolds and Miss America contestants from the 1960s to the late 1980s and found that, although the models got progressively thinner, their waist-to-hip ratios remained exactly the same, with their waists reliably measuring between 68 per cent and 72 per cent of the size of their hips: a ratio Singh expresses as 'WHRs of 0.68 to 0.72'. But was this something peculiar to the West, or could it be a more universal phenomenon? To try to find out, Singh made outline drawings of twelve women, four of whom were thin, four average-sized and four relatively heavy. He then manipulated their waist-to-hip ratios so that some were very low and some very high and asked 580 people of different ages, races, and cultural backgrounds to rate the women on the basis of attractiveness.

By far the most popular was the medium-sized woman with the lowest waist-to-hip ratio. Second was the medium-sized woman with the second lowest WHR, but as women from the lighter and heavier groups began to enter the ratings, it was clear that they were being ordered not on the basis of their weight, but according to their WHRs. Thus, a heavy woman with a low WHR was considered universally more attractive than a medium-sized woman with a high WHR. People reported that she not only looked more attractive, she also seemed more youthful and, crucially, more fertile too.

When Singh's drawings were taken out of America and shown around the world, the effect was even more striking. From Hong Kong to India, from Africa to the Azores, people varied according to how heavy they liked their women, but they varied not a jot in the waist-to-hip ratio they preferred. Always, it was the smallest. As if to drive the point home further, when the drawings were shown to one of the remotest tribes on Earth, the Shiwiar of the Amazonian rainforest, the men volunteered information on the fertility of the women without even being asked. Pointing to a medium-sized woman with a very low waist-to-hip ratio one tribesman remarked: 'This is the most beautiful. She can have six or eight children.' Pointing to a less curvaceous one, he added, 'This other one can't have as many.'

To these men, totally uninfluenced by Western standards, there was a direct and explicit correlation between attractiveness, a low waist-to-hip ratio and the ability to have children – a correlation which Singh feels is embedded in the mind of every man to help him find, and fall for, the most reproductively viable mates. In support of his theory, a study from Holland has recently reported that among women undergoing in vitro fertilisation, those with the lowest WHRs have by far the largest chance of conceiving. Indeed, for every 10 per cent increase in WHR, the chance of conceiving drop by 30 per cent.

The perfect average

A well-proportioned body, lustrous hair and fine, pellucid skin. These three easily observable, clearly demonstrable attributes have always served as reliable guides to an individual's youth, fitness and fertility. And although all three apply in some degree to men as well – whose waist-to-hip ratio should be between 80 and 90 per cent, who should strive to be as tall as possible (one recent report from the Wall Street Journal suggested that every inch in height is worth another $6,000 per year in salary), and who should seek to retain as much of their hair as late into life as possible – physical attributes such as these are relatively insignificant for men when compared to other, less visible cues like status and resources. However, when one gets close up, a plethora of other signals come into play, signals which apply equally to both men and women, and which are etched into the lines and contours of that most expressive of fertility billboards: the face.

In the late nineteenth century, Sir Francis Galton, a distinguished scientist, cousin of Charles Darwin, and a notorious racist, determined to construct the ultimate criminal face by taking photographic portraits of a number of crooks and villains and superimposing them one on top of the other. The result, he felt, could be used to identify likely criminals and stop them from breeding a class of incorrigible and hopeless felons. Unfortunately, when he blended all the faces together he found that, instead of producing the gothically crooked mask he had hoped to create, the special villainous irregularities he had collected had actually averaged each other out to create a bland yet curiously attractive composite.

Exactly a century later, the same technique is being used by Judith Langlois and her team at the University of Texas to test our perceptions of beauty. By feeding many faces into her computer programme, she is able to create an overall template, a perfect average, which she then shows to colleagues, students, and friends. Invariably, they agree that the composite face is superior to all the individual faces. Langlois believes not only that we are born with the capacity to detect beauty, but that our beauty detectors are calibrated to respond to a sort of ideal face, which we either average out very early in life or which may even be implanted in us before birth. To see whether this might be true, she has tested previously rated attractive and unattractive faces both on people from different cultures and backgrounds, and on very young children, who have had much less opportunity to acquire a culturally based concept of beauty. Not only do all ethnicities agree on who is more beautiful, the babies agree too, spending much more time looking at the beautiful faces, and playing for longer periods of time with beautifully faced dolls.

Langlois' research is intriguing, but her finding that whatever is most average is most attractive has met with some resistance from other facial experts who suggest that, although averageness is helpful, it's not the whole story. The faces that we find truly beautiful, they suggest, are average faces which have been manipulated in certain key dimensions: jaw-size, chin-size, and brow-size.

Victor Johnston in particular, at New Mexico State University, has devised a game called Faceprints, which can be accessed on the Internet by visiting his web-site.* In one version players are shown thirty faces, all male or all female, which they are asked to rate on a beauty scale of one to nine. The top-rated faces are then bred with one another to create

* http://www-psych.nmsu.edu/~vic/faceprints/

two digital offspring, which replace the lowest-rated faces in the pool. Gradually, the faces evolve to become more and more attractive, until a player finally gives one face a perfect ten and the game stops. Johnston then compares the average of all the first-generation faces to the ideal ten which has signalled the end of the game. In the case of males, he habitually finds that the ideal has a larger jaw, a stronger chin and a more imposing brow than the average. In the case of females, the reverse is true, with a small jaw being particularly prized, as well as a long, flat upper face with prominent eyes and cheekbones.

The reason for these preferences, believes Johnston, is that the brow, chin and cheekbones are precisely the areas which are most affected by the rush of testosterone and oestrogen which signals puberty. A high forehead and small chin are, in effect, markers of a high oestrogen surge which, in women, is associated with high fertility. Similarly, the broad lower jaw of the male signals a healthy rush of testosterone, which would have been good news, in our ancestral environment, for females seeking strength and protection. Testosterone, in fact, is a doubly effective marker of reproductive potential since, as well as generating size and strength, it adversely affects the immune system, obliging the body to regulate the amount it produces so as not to exceed safe dosages, except during brief periods of pubertal acne. As a result, if an individual has a strong brow, a large lower jaw and well-developed shoulders, he is advertising his immunity to disease as well as his overall virility.

Cheerful symmetry

Together with Langlois' theory of averageness and Johnston's theory of extremes, the third major cornerstone of research into facial beauty perception is being investigated by Randy Thornhill at the University of New Mexico in Albuquerque.

Thornhill, a behavioural ecologist who spent the first two decades of his professional life studying the sex life of the Japanese scorpionfly, turned his attention to humans during the mid-1980s, fascinated to discover whether some of his findings about our winged brethren might apply to our own species as well. Particularly interesting in Thornhill's mind was the potential link between symmetry and sexiness. Among scorpion flies, those with the most symmetrical body parts, judged by the extent to which their left and right sides matched, were much the most effective in attracting and retaining mates. This they appeared able to achieve even when they were hidden from view, using a pheromone which their potential lovers could smell but not see.

To investigate whether the same sort of judgements might be made by humans, Thornhill assembled several hundred students from his university and set about measuring their symmetry across seven different dimensions: feet, ankles, hands, wrists, elbows and breadth and length of ears. He then issued those students with a confidential question-naire asking when they lost their virginity, how many sex partners they had had, and much more besides. When Thornhill analysed the results with his colleague Steve Gangestad, a very clear picture began to emerge. Not only had the most symmetrical males lost their vir-ginity on average three to four years earlier than their more lopsided bedfellows, symmetry was also an accurate predictor of sexual suc-cess, with the most symmetrical members of either sex having experi-enced not just an earlier start but a much greater number of part-ners.

And this was only the beginning. In a later study, Thornhill and Gangestad produced a finding – as yet unreplicated – that highly sym-metrical men were likely to give women more orgasms (a finding which ties in eerily well with Baker and Bellis's ideas about female infidelity), and that they may be more intelligent as well. Similarly, information is emerging from the University of Michigan that the most symmetrical members of either sex may also be the most healthy, reporting fewer outbreaks of every sort of upset from nasal congestion and insomnia through to jealousy and rage.

In our ancestral environment, when the adaptation for preferring sym-metrical individuals would have developed, much of the body would have been on view, and every part might have provided some clue about its owner's reproductive fitness. For example, Thornhill and Gangestad have also found that symmetrical breasts tally with greater fertility, that sym-metrical figures testify to developmental stability, and that symmetrical faces indicate well-mixed genes and excellent parasite immunity. But there's still much more to be discovered about symmetry; and it may turn out to have unexpected subtleties. In one remarkable study, John Manning from the University of Liverpool has shown that female facial symmetry may subtly increase around ovulation through a process of soft tissue swelling, making women marginally more attractive just when they are most fertile.

Scents and sensibility

If our eyes have been made particularly sensitive to beauty, many would say that our noses have become less so. As our ancestors learned to walk upright, the better to shade their bodies from the scorching African sun, our eyes could see further but our noses lost the plot. Scents which had been deposited by ourselves and other animals to mark our territory or track our routes, slipped out of our everyday perception and slid into the chambers of our subconscious, forgotten and all but forgone.

This, at least, is what might have happened. Indeed, many of us imagine that it actually has happened. After all, we pride ourselves on being a more or less odourless society, scrubbing and sluicing until our more recognisable body odours are extinguished, and then replacing them with commercially produced and often warring substitutes: roses, cloves, sandalwood, citrus, jasmine.

Yet behind these baroque constructions, perfumers hold a secret. The most expensive elements in any perfume, whether for men or women, are not taken from fruit, flowers, or spices, but from the nether regions of other animals: musk, from the belly of the musk deer, ambergris from the gut of the sperm whale, civet from the anal scent glands of wild Ethiopian tomcats, castoreum from the rear end of the beaver. Gathered at great expense, and often illegally, from an ever-diminishing collection of animals, these notes are what give scents their sensual flavour, their sex appeal, their raw base power. We may notice the fruit, but we react to the animal.

Should we rid ourselves of perfume and aftershave and allow our bodies to breathe and exhale, we would soon find that our natural odours returned, perhaps less potent than they were among our ancestors, but potent nonetheless. Their smells have been described in the factual arena by individuals like Helen Keller, who, deprived of sight and hearing, found her olfactory abilities greatly enhanced, and in the fictional world by characters like Grenouille, the villain at the centre of Patrick Süskind's novel *Perfume*. Grenouille is an eighteenth-century chemist who, determined to anoint himself with the most seductive and irresistible smell

THE SEXUAL SELF

Cartoon by R. Chast for the *New Yorker* magazine, printed shortly after the discovery of the 'gay gene' had been announced.

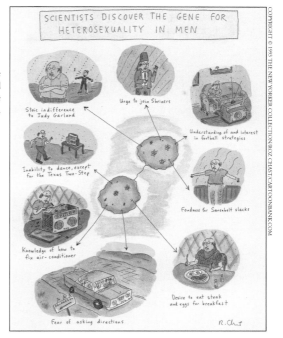

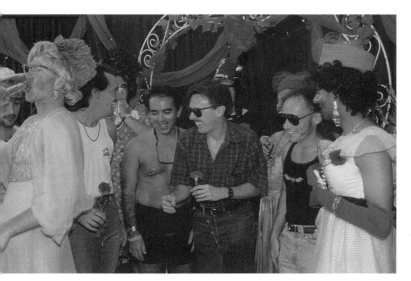

queens at a Gay Pride rally. Could gender identity really be inscribed in the brain?

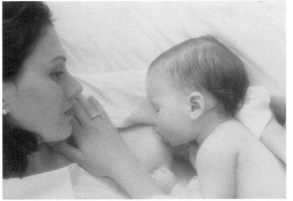

A breastfeeding mother. The way she relates to her baby may profoundly influence its own attachment styles later in life.

Gender play: boys tend to gravitate towards 'masculine' and aggressive toys like trucks and guns.

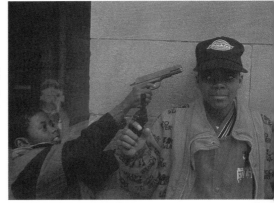

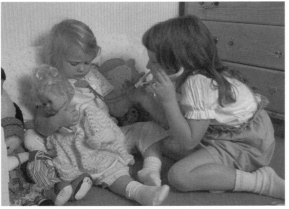

Girls, meanwhile, prefer dolls and more 'inclusive' activities. But how much of this behaviour is inborn and how much learned as children grow up?

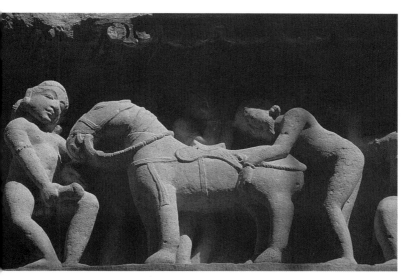

...ality has been a part of sexual experimentation in many cultures. It is graphically illustrated in ...ngs on the Lakshmana temple in Khajuraho, India.

Elaborations on the basic theme: small ads from a men's porn magazine.

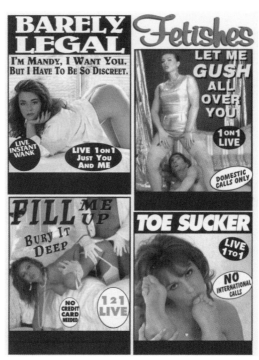

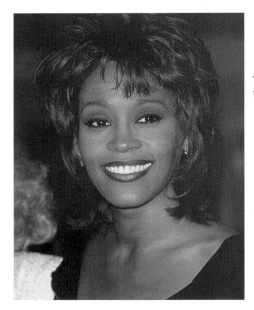

Whitney Houston –
the most beautiful woman in the worl

The young Marlon Brando –
the most handsome man?

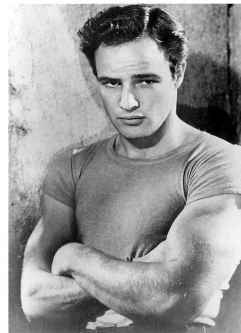

'36–24–36': study of waist-to-hip ratio in women by Devendra Singh. Singh found a direct correlation between low waist-to-hip ratios, attractiveness and the ability to bear children – all over the world.

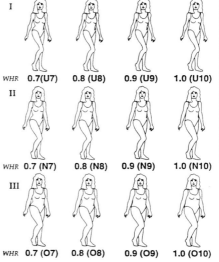

I			
WHR 0.7(U7)	0.8 (U8)	0.9 (U9)	1.0 (U10)
II			
WHR 0.7 (N7)	0.8 (N8)	0.9 (N9)	1.0 (N10)
III			
WHR 0.7 (O7)	0.8 (O8)	0.9 (O9)	1.0 (O10)

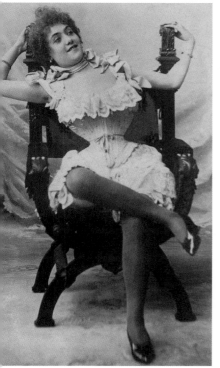

Waist-to-hip ratio taken to its extreme: a severe corset from the mid-nineteenth century.

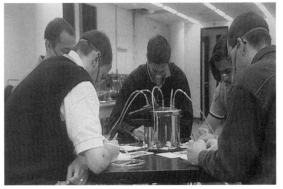

Men inhale female copulin[e]
an experiment by Astrid Jü[t]
It demonstrates the importa[nce]
of odour as one of the mos[t]
sophisticated and subtle of [our]
sexual signalling systems.

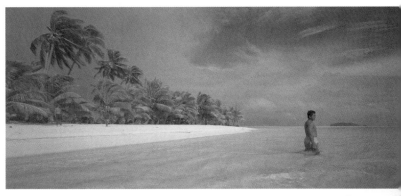

Mangaia, southernmost of [the]
Cook Islands. Was this a p[lace]
devoted to pleasure yet de[void]
of romantic attachment?
Or merely an illustration [of]
the West's obsession with [it?]

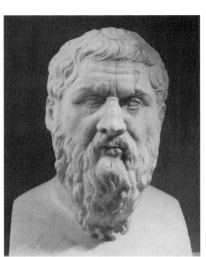

Plato, one of the most influential
of the ancient Greek philosophers,
who pictured love as an incredibly
finely-tuned mechanism which
inspired us to seek, recognise
and respond to the very person
with whom we truly deserved
to be joined.

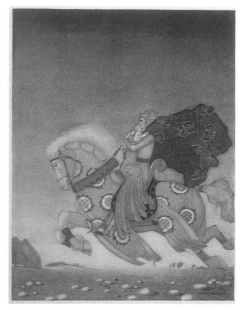

Tristan and Isolde: one of the great romantic myths of the Western world.

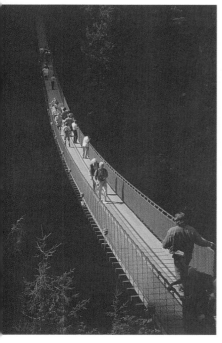

The Capilano suspension bridge near Vancouver: scene of an unusual experiment by Donald Dutton and Art Aron, who tried to prove the importance of anxiety in sexual attraction.

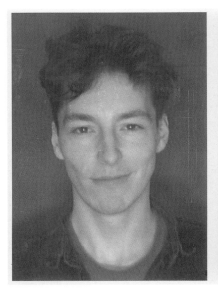
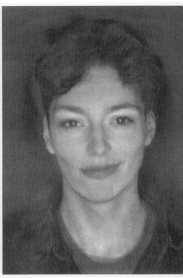

Intriguing evidence for the Narcissus effect. When shown various faces, people sometimes choose a sex-changed version of their own as the most attractive.

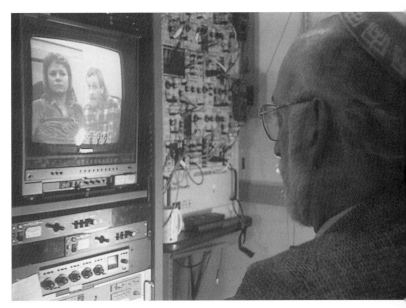

Marriage counselling, the modern way. Psychologist John Gottman observes as a couple discuss an area of continuing conflict in their marriage while wired up to an array of technological equipment he knows, takes to murdering young virgins and extracting their natural odours with wax compresses.

Perfume is a cautionary tale about personal and sexual obsessiveness, and its gothic construction and highly tuned prose brings the reader's nose alive to nuances of smell of which we are rarely consciously aware. Not just the general human odour, 'a sweaty-oily, sour-cheesy, quite richly repulsive basic theme' that clung to all humans equally in earlier times, but the very specific individual odours of babies, children, men and women, all of whom smell subtly different at different ages, in different moods, and at different times of the month.

At about the time Süskind was writing *Perfume*, Karl Grammer (who conducted the night-club study mentioned in Chapter 2) was working with his postgraduate students on a seminal series of studies in exactly this territory: the nature of male and female odours, and the ways in which they might affect our social and sexual desires.

In one study, Grammer set out to investigate male odours, in particular how women might be attracted to or repelled by them, depending on where they themselves were in their menstrual cycle. Grammer's own work in the night-club, as well as Baker and Bellis's work, suggested that around ovulation, women might be open to sensations and experiences which would otherwise interest them much less. Starting from the blunt premise that 'men do indeed stink', Grammer invited 290 women to sniff a cloth pad steeped in one of the principal ingredients of male sweat: androstenon. They had to say what the smell reminded them of and whether they rated it positively or negatively. They then had to give some personal information about their age, whether they took the Pill, and what point they were at in their menstrual cycles.

Androstenon research had been going on for some time, and had already thrown up some suggestive results. When British researchers had sprayed chairs or telephone booths with it, they found that women – and occasionally men – would occupy them for longer. Androstenon was a principal player in the sexy, seductive smells of musky perfumes and of the gourmet's delight, truffles. But androstenon was a double-edged sword, seeming to carry as many overtones of aggression or unpleasantness as of sexiness, especially to other men. One commercial odour-research firm had found that bills scented with it were likely to be paid quicker. And Grammer's sniffers, when asked to identify the smell on the pads, came up with some pretty unflattering free-associations:

sweat, urine, glue, chemistry sets, 'men on the pull'. The overall rating of androstenon was overwhelmingly negative. If male smell was such a turn-off, Grammer wondered, how on earth might it be to men's sexual benefit to have evolved it?

The key to the puzzle emerged when Grammer linked the women's responses to the smell of androstenon with where they were in their menstrual cycles. Those who were ovulating had given much more positive descriptions of the smell, and their overall ratings were neutral, compared to the negative reactions of the whole sample. The message was clear: male smell didn't attract women; rather, it acted as a kind of ovulation radar, allowing men to get further with women who were ovulating and fertile.

At the same time, Grammer's postgraduate student Astrid Jütte was investigating female odours, and finding some equally Machiavellian processes. Jütte synthesised mixtures of chemicals to mimic the smell of the vaginal secretions of women at various stages in their monthly cycles, and stored them in stainless steel pots which could then be sniffed by randomly selected male raters. As each man smelled one of the mixtures, dubbed copulines, he was asked to look at and rate photographs of different women, evaluating their attractiveness. There were four different mixtures: one contained the odour of menstruating women; one was more like ovulating women; one resembled premenstrual women, and the fourth was just water.

The results were intricate but intriguing. The highest-rated smell, by default, was water since the men generally found the other odours unpleasant. However, these very same 'unpleasant' odours actually made men's ratings of the photographs rise. Moreover, the effect was strongest with women who weren't all that impressive visually. Photographs rated ordinary or only mildly attractive when the men were smelling water were reported as being quite or very attractive when they were smelling copulines. What's more, the copuline mix mimicking that of ovulating women made the men's testosterone levels soar, pushing them up in some instances by 150 per cent. Although the men weren't consciously finding the smells attractive, their odour detectors were in direct communication with their subconscious, bypassing the decision-making process and instructing them at the deepest, most direct level, to forget their reserve and follow their noses.

Grammer and Jütte's experiments suggest that despite the perceived unimportance of human odour, it is actually one of the most sophisticated and subtle of our sexual signalling systems, able to distinguish not just generally suitable candidates for copulation but precise windows of time during which it should most fruitfully occur. Yet although their work is intriguing, perhaps the most remarkable odour-based experiment has been conducted over the border from their Viennese labs, in Switzerland.

Wedekind the wunderkind

In a complex of magnificent buildings on the bustling, prosperous streets of Bern, thousands of students from all over Europe race to their lectures. The solid, self-reliant, work ethic of the University of Bern might seem a world apart from the fleshpots of Vienna, Amsterdam and Munich, where much of the most sophisticated European sex research takes place, but it's been hitting the headlines since the early 1990s, when biology whizzkid Claus Wedekind started using it as his base to examine the effect on mate selection of what is known as 'the major histo-compatibility complex'. In short, he wanted to know whether we can smell our perfect partner. Not just any partner, but the right partner for us. Even to his students, this seemed like an impossible task. It was hard enough to believe that we could detect the odour of fertility, let alone the odour of compatibility. How could such an odour exist? What would it smell like?

To find out, Wedekind assembled a group of men and asked them to wear a single T-shirt for two successive nights, and to abstain from the usual list of odour-producing activities, including aftershave use, garlic eating and sex. The T-shirts were then coded and placed in boxes with only a small triangular hole at the top. A selection of women were then invited into the labs to place their noses in the boxes and inhale. To gee up their olfactory acuity, Wedekind had provided each of them with two presents, one pharmacological and one literary. The pharmacological one was a nasal spray that supported the regeneration of their mucous membranes and made sure their sense of smell wasn't smothered by congestion. The literary one was a copy of *Perfume*, to render them more aware of the possible permutations of odour.

As the women wafted the male odours into their nostrils, they were asked to rate each T-shirt for intensity, pleasantness and sexiness. So far, this doesn't sound markedly different from the experiments by Grammer and Jütte, but there was one crucial difference. Whereas Grammer and

Jütte had been working on the assumption that all men smelled roughly the same, Wedekind was looking for differences. In fact, he was looking for differences in one very specific area. As well as being tested for their odours, the men had all been required to give a blood sample so that researchers could map a part of their individual genetic make-up. Among the tens of thousands of genes possessed by every individual, there are three small groups which code for our immunity to different diseases. These are the genes which make up the major histo-compatibility complex, known as the MHC. And in Wedekind's experiment, it wasn't just the men who were required to give blood samples, it was the women too.

From a purely genetic point of view, the sturdiest, most disease-resistant children would be likely to be born to couples who had different genes on their MHC configurations. Different genes would mean resistance to different diseases. A mixed combination of different resistance patterns would be good news for any child who inherited them. From a purely genetic point of view, therefore, it would make sense to be more attracted to people with different MHC configurations than to people with the same ones as yourself. But could our sense of smell be so finely tuned, so perfectly calibrated, as to recognise and respond to the odours of individual genes? It seemed impossible, but that was Wedekind's finding.

Nearly every woman judged the smell of men whose MHC complexes were different from her own as stronger, more pleasant, and considerably sexier too. When Wedekind announced his results, he was met with incredulity and amazement in equal proportions. His e-mail was log-jammed, his telephone never stopped ringing, and he was obliged to spend the first few months after he announced his results fielding interview requests from newspapers and magazines in more than thirty countries.

Why are we so interested? What's so amazing about smelling other people's genes? And even if we have the power to do so, surely it doesn't influence our mate choice in the swirling, complex cauldron of real life? Wedekind, believe it or not, thinks it does. And so do his volunteers. For when the experiment was over and the women were asked to reflect on their day, many recalled that they were struck by one particular thought. The smells they enjoyed were preferred not only because they seemed the most pleasing, but also because they were strangely redolent of the women's own boyfriends or ex-boyfriends. Presumably, it's possible that the association with past or present partners might have influenced the women's enjoyment of the smells — but it's also possible that the smells had played a role, however subtle, in their choice of partners in the first place.

This then is the true secret of Wedekind's study. From all the millions of people we encounter in our lifetime, from all the coincidences that are thrown in our path and from all the choices we make, our minds and the bodies they inhabit may have the capacity to narrow down our patterns of desire beyond the basic human need for variety, beyond the scripts within which our culture permits us to operate. Beyond even the people our upbringing obliges us to admire, to the one type of person, even to the one individual, who may be 'made for us' in a special, almost literal way.

If so, then surely we should know as much about these powers as possible, for they might hold the key to the one thing for which we search beyond all else. Our soulmate, our loved one. The perfect partner. Our other half. It is that search, and the criteria we use to engage in it, that the next chapter investigates.

6

Falling in Love

Little Green was the most beautiful girl in the camp. With her braided hair and hand-embroidered knickers, she put all the other girls to shame. She danced in the dormitories, sang in the fields, and had an unusually sprightly gait, as if she felt the world more intensely, more vibrantly than the others with whom she shared her life.

The year was 1974. The place, the Red Fire Farm near the shore of the East China Sea. These were the years of Mao's most iron-clad dictatorship, when the Little Red Book was read and revered across the nation, when the arias from Madame Mao's revolutionary operas filled the theatres, homes and fields and where Communist slogans like 'The Party is great, glorious and correct!' and 'We would rather have socialist weeds than capitalist crops!' were spoken, nay shouted, with burning zeal.

The Red Fire Farm was one of a number of large agrarian co-operatives where young men and women were sent to labour for the People's Republic, picking wheat, cotton and oil-bearing seeds from dawn till dusk, their ears filled with propaganda and their feet caked with mud. At the end of a long day's work, they returned from the fields exhausted and, after a bowl of rice, fell straight to sleep. Here, they dreamed of the Revolution, of the glorious visage of their Chairman, of victory over the capitalists. But here, Little Green dreamed of love.

Some weeks previously, she had met a comrade from a neighbouring farm, a young, bookish man in glasses. When she returned to her bunk she had been unable to get him out of her mind. He was reasonably tall, reasonably handsome. But there was more to him than that. Something unknown. Something almost indescribable. He fitted something inside of her; a dream, an image she carried in her head. The two of them together living out their life in each other's company. Happy, contented. In love. Of all the people she had ever met, of all the people she was ever likely to meet, this was the man for her. And she yearned for him with a desire which was quite unlike her love for Mao, for her country, for the life she had so far led. And she knew that her desire was wrong. Lately, the *People's Daily* and the *Red Flag*, the state-sanctioned newspapers and magazines, had been cracking down on adult relationships. Flirting, courting, dating – all these activities were considered frivolous, unnecessary, wasteful. They took up time which could be better spent furthering the cause of the Revolution. And worst of all, they detracted from absolute loyalty to Mao. This was why, on Red Fire Farm at least, romantic love between two people had been banned.

Little Green was afraid of what would happen if she and her lover were caught together. Afraid of being punished, of being humiliated. But most of all, afraid of being separated. That was why the two lovers met in secret. By night, out in the furthest fields, under the wide canopy of the stars. It was the most romantic thing in the world.

Then, one night in early summer, as Little Green and her lover were together in the fields, they heard a rustling. They turned around. At first, they saw nothing. Then, suddenly, a flashlight came on. Then another. Then another. Soon, they were caught in the beams of more than thirty torches. The rest of the camp had heard about their activities and been summoned to apprehend them. At the head of the delegation was the camp commandant, Yan.

Yan decided to make an example of the pair. Little Green was brain-washed into signing a document which accused her lover of raping her; he was swiftly executed. Little Green was sent back to her camp, shamed, and told not to fall in love again. From that moment on, she stopped singing and ceased to braid her hair. Her underpants became torn and she no longer embroidered them. Slowly, in front of her comrades, she sank into despair. No one could comfort or console her. She became bloated, dirty. She withdrew into herself completely. Her eyes looked dead and she no longer spoke. A few months later, she was found face down, floating in the river. Unable to be with her lover in life, she had joined him in death.

Anchee Min, a former Red Guard and propaganda-film actress who tells Little Green's story in her autobiography, *Red Azalea*, saw at first hand the destructive, stultifying power of an ideology which refuses to accept romantic love as a real or worthwhile phenomenon. Mao may have been the most recent person to espouse this point of view, feeling that it was as unnecessary as it was unhelpful, but he was by no means the only one. For throughout its long and chequered history, love (and what to do about it) has been the subject of more stories and plays, more myths and legends, more tracts and documents, than any other human emotion. Praised by some as the pinnacle of human existence and by others as the source of all misery, love is perhaps the most debated yet least understood of all the human emotions.

Certainly, love poses a disturbing number of questions. While it might be vital for parental care, it's certainly not necessary for reproduction. It's not the same thing as lust, or admiration, or even affection. It's not essential for workable – or even for pleasurable – sexual relationships or marriage. And different societies, it emerges, have indeed treated romantic love in wholly different ways. Depending on where and when a man or woman lives, it might either be apparently beyond their emotional horizons, or at the very centre of their universe.

Anthropologists who fanned out across the world during the middle years of this century always came back with contradictory stories. There were the Mangaians of the South Pacific, who were so lusty they had no need for romantic love. There were the Ik of East Africa, who were so sad and desperate that they had forgotten how to feel it. At the other extreme there were the writers of ancient Sanskrit texts, who were so acutely aware of all its power and permutations that they had more than twenty different words for it.

Indeed, there were so many views about whether love existed, what it was, why it arose, how it felt, what should be done about it, that it seemed as if everyone were talking about a slightly different experience. There were common points, to be sure. Everyone agreed it could be powerful. Everyone agreed that it could strike suddenly, almost without warning. But as soon as one tried to examine it, it began to slip through the fingers; it was just too delicate to be entrapped, too subtle to succumb, too elusive to be captured by a phrase and pinned, like a butterfly, to a label with its kingdom, phylum, class, order, family, genus and species.

This is partly why, in the mid-1970s, the American Senator William Proxmire scotched an application for state funding into research on romantic love in the United States, suggesting that any attempts to understand it in all but the most passing and poetical of fashions were ridiculous. In an interview with *Time* magazine, he was quoted as saying

'I believe that 200 million other Americans want to leave some things in life a mystery, and right at the top of things we don't want to know is why a man falls in love with a woman and vice versa. Even if they could give us an answer, we wouldn't want to hear it.'

As a result of his comments, thousands of dollars' worth of state funding of the nascent research into romantic love, aimed at understanding one of the most perplexing mysteries in the human psyche, was cut. The academic world fell silent. Was it because they agreed with the Senator's verdict, or was it because they were retreating only to regroup, considering how best to approach such an elusive and apparently sacrosanct prey?

From love to limerence

The drive from Washington DC to Rehoboth Beach takes one across the glassy waters of Chesapeake Bay and down through the marshy flats of Delaware. To the left is the grey swell of the Atlantic. To the right, an endless expanse of shining, crop-filled fields. It's a beautiful but rather eerie landscape, with only an occasional clapboard house rising from the dead flat of the horizon. In one of these low, snug houses, just by a small junction, lives a quiet, middle-aged lady with a choirboy haircut and a slight limp. Her name is Dorothy Tennov.

Tennov, who for fifteen years has scarcely left her house, is just starting to get out and about again. She plays the piano for her local Brethren church, teaches part time at the Academy for Lifelong Learning (a sort of university for the over-sixties) and has just started taking up her pen to write again. Yet despite her usual reclusivity, brought on by a row with the University of Bridgeport, where she used to hold a chair in experimental psychology, Tennov has made one of the greatest contributions to love research this century. If Lawrence and Auden wrote about it, and Russell and Barthes philosophised about it, Tennov has tried to define it. Her goal was not to enter the psychology textbooks, although she has, and not to gain fame, which she also has. Rather, it was to help her students. They were capable, to be sure; some of them were brilliant. Yet it wasn't their academic lives with which Tennov was trying to help: it was their personal lives, and in particular, their love lives.

Tennov recalls that the idea to investigate love came to her one day when a student named Marilyn failed to hand in some coursework on time. When Tennov asked her why, she suddenly burst into tears, sobbing through her handkerchief that she had just been discarded by her boyfriend Mark, whom she had hoped to marry and with whom she was still completely smitten. Mark had written her a rejection letter just two days before and she had been unable to think about anything since. Her world had fallen apart. The rug had been pulled from underneath her feet. Her future, once so bright, now seemed to stop dead just in front of her.

Tennov took pity, but instead of simply excusing her and going back to other business, she began to think. How many of her other students had been through this sort of agony? Who, in her class, in her course, in her university, were in the throes of love affairs which, whether happy or sad, were occupying their every waking thought, interfering with their lives, altering their moods and personalities? And if it was widespread in her university, exerting effects on the day-to-day lives of her students, how much havoc must it wreak in the real world? Was this really a topic that didn't merit, or couldn't support, further investigation?

Tennov decided to issue a questionnaire, first to her students, then to anyone who would listen. She wanted to know whether there was any common ground between Marilyn's experiences and those of her other students, and between those of her other students and the rest of her respondents. If so, perhaps she could start to identify the special components of falling in love, the better to understand the condition, the better to appraise its causes, components and effects.

Her answers, coded and processed in her book *Love and Limerence: The Experience of Being in Love*, represent the first formal attempt in modern times to strip love down to its component parts, and examine their structure and function. What she produced was both a working definition of love and a state which was so distinct, so crystalline, that she decided to honour it with a term all it own: 'limerence'. This state, wrote Tennov, had been experienced at one time or another by more than 98 per cent of her respondents, and was remarkable both for its consistency and predictability. It was a more specific state than 'love', roughly equivalent to what we variously describe as 'falling in love', 'being head over heels', or 'going crazy' for someone. It was that exhilarating, urgent, overbearing rush of feeling one just couldn't ignore. Tennov outlined the major components of limerence, and set them down so that people could understand not just the characteristics of the condition but also its course.

Most of Tennov's five hundred respondents could pinpoint the exact moment when the whole experience began. Sometimes it started with a shared conversation, sometimes with a stolen glance. Sometimes the individual in question was an old friend, sometimes a new acquaintance. Whatever the circumstances, and whoever the person, the distinguishing characteristic of the first incident was simply that they suddenly started to take on a new and special significance – a significance which would make them, for a time at least, the most important person in the world.

One of Tennov's respondents, a university professor called Dr Vesteroy, described the moment well. He had just finished holding a faculty meeting and was turning to leave when he noticed that one of his younger staff members, a Dr Ashton, had remained behind. He writes:

Suddenly, Dr Ashton – Elena, her name is – looked up and seemed startled to find herself the only leftover from the meeting. She flushed a bit and gathered her things, saying that she hoped she had not kept me. Then just before she went out, she looked at me and smiled! It was that smile and that look that started the whole thing off . . . I had this flash, this thrill, a running sensation of excitement, and I don't even remember what I said . . . some spark of communication had passed between us and it was communication of a very personal and delightful sort.

Once the spark has been ignited, Tennov notes, the lover feels a surge of excitement, a burst of energy, and a heightened sense of well-being. The chance of true happiness is in the air. A great sense of freedom, of infinite possibilities. Any such feelings are, however, fleeting, for no sooner have they started than they are accompanied by sudden bursts of Tennov's second major characteristic: intrusive thinking.

Gently at first, and then with increasing force and frequency, the loved one starts to impinge on the lover's thoughts. The lover imagines what the loved one is doing, what they are feeling, what they would think of the book they are reading, the clothes they are wearing, their parents, pastimes, and friends. Tennov asked her study group to estimate how much time they spent thinking about their loved one, and while answers varied between 30 per cent and 100 per cent, everyone conceded that such thoughts had an involuntary, almost obsessive quality about them.

However much you tried to put your loved one out of your mind, the
kept on coming back.

Accompanying these constant imaginings, of course, is the lover'
urgent hope that the loved one will reciprocate their desire. Yet, ii
the initial stages of love, Tennov writes that complete reciprocatio
is not as powerful a fuel as some element of delay, some componen
of denial. This, she suggests, is what creates the aching of the hear
the intense yearning, the complete dependency of mood and apparen
subjection of the lover to the beloved. It is also what makes the love
pick over every detail of the most recent meeting – from what the love
was wearing to the words they spoke, the intonation they used, and th
look which accompanied them – searching for signs which might indicat
the possibility of reciprocation and, therefore, the promise of paradise. D
Vesteroy was particularly prone to this sort of second-guessing, this sor
of obsessive anatomising of meetings in the early stages of his relationshi
with Dr Ashton. He writes:

> Despite all logic, I could not shake off the feeling – the hope
> as well – that Elena's totally circumspect behaviour was itself an
> indication that her feelings were not unlike my own. How could
> she know that my wife and I were having marital difficulties? Her
> very circumspection became proof of inner turmoil . . . At first I'd
> set up little tests. I'd say that if at the next meeting she elects to sit
> beside me or facing me, I will count it as proof that this madness
> is not unilateral. But when she chose a seat farthest from me, or
> one which made it very difficult for us to look at one another, I
> realised that the test was not a test at all. No matter what she did,
> I could interpret it in my favour. Her remote position in the room
> could serve the function of helping her to hide feelings as intense as
> my own. She was as afraid as I was of overt interaction!

The incredible importance which every meeting takes on naturall
makes them as terrifying as they are exciting. Vesteroy, increasingl
obsessed with every passing day, writes: 'My mind was filled with her, m
knees trembled when I saw her, and I fashioned all manner of elaborat
schemes whereby I could test the ground before taking a step. I felt
had to do something, but I was completely paralysed by fear that th
whole affair existed only in my imagination and that I would mak

an utter fool of myself and destroy any chance of success that might possibly exist.'

In the initial stages of limerence, Tennov writes that it is feasible to desire several people at a time, but at the magical moment when reciprocation first occurs, all other contenders are shut out, and the experience takes on an intensity and exclusivity that marks it out from all other styles of relationship. Here, although sexual attraction is almost always strong, the lover is also aware that they are feeling something more special, something more spiritual; something from the depths of their soul as well as from the core of their body.

While the hapless Vesteroy continued to plot and pine, another of Tennov's respondents, this time a student, was a little more successful. Having enjoyed her first night with her lover, she wrote, 'My delight in simply existing eclipsed everything else, and I literally could scarcely feel the ground as I walked. In some ways, my perceptions grew stronger. Colours seemed more brilliant. The warmth of the sunlight on my arm as I drove to work was so acutely pleasurable that I marvelled at never before appreciating it.' Following the lead of Simone de Beauvoir, Tennov's informant describes this state as one of 'ecstatic union', and it is usually accompanied by another of the great distinguishing characteristics of limerence; something which Tennov (this time borrowing from Stendhal) calls 'crystallisation'.

Stendhal, the nineteenth-century French novelist best known for his epic *Le Rouge et le Noir*, also wrote a tract on romantic love in which he drew attention to the sort of shimmering, bejewelled magnificence which the loved one takes on in the eyes of the beloved, such that they appear to have no faults, only an endless array of charming, precious, almost perfect qualities. Stendhal dubbed this process crystallisation, after a process he had observed in the salt mines of Hallein, near Salzburg. If you threw a stick into the waters by these mines, just an ordinary common-or-garden stick, and left it for a few weeks, by the time you returned it would have accreted a large number of shimmering salt crystals all over its surface. Shining, glistening, sparkling in the light, it no longer appeared like a stick, but like a jewelled wand; something magical, almost mystical. You would now be blind to the fact that it was a stick and open only to the possibility that it was something of rare and great value; something of unrivalled beauty.

Tennov, much influenced by Stendhal, agrees that crystallisation is an integral part of limerence, but perceives its effect rather differently. Instead of the crystals obscuring the loved one's faults and replacing them with diamonds, Tennov believes that the faults themselves become diamonds. In this scheme of things, the lover can perceive the loved one's shortcomings just as clearly as the next person, they just interpret them differently. Whereas for most people, a wart is a wart is a wart, for the lover looking at the beloved, a wart is both cute and adorable. Furthermore, while ignoring or even admiring the faults of the loved one, the lover also greatly exaggerates their positive qualities, so that a tendency toward kindness is seen as an enormous generosity of soul, and a pair of beautiful blue eyes become the bluest and most beautiful that ever were seen.

By these and other methods, the loved one acquires an even greater magnificence in the eyes of the lover. As a result, the reciprocation for which the lover so ardently longs seems even more improbable but when given, leads to even greater joy. Uncertainty, sensitivity and longing are heightened even more, creating a sort of spiral which can only be broken by complete and enduring reciprocation or by utter contempt and abandonment. In the former case, a more realistic, enduring attachment can start to develop. In the latter, despair, either temporary or permanent, takes hold.

This, then, represents the complete set of behaviours, emotions and cognitions which between them, were reported by almost all of Tennov's respondents and which made up the full experience of limerence. It was a process that was deeply disruptive, that was often as disturbing as it was delightful, and which many reported as having been the most gut-wrenching experience in their lives. Could something as profound and apparently constant as this simply be an invention of the West?

For all Tennov's powers of description, and for all the power of the process she had described, there were indeed societies which seemed to have none of these shimmering visions. Societies where couples met and married for money, duty or children, where men and women lived separate lives without a hint of 'romance'. Now that love and limerence had been defined, it was time to test them in other periods and places.

Coming of age on Mangaia

When Helen Harris's tiny plane touched down on Mangaia, she knew little of what to expect. There were numerous guide books to the Pacific islands, but most concentrated, not surprisingly, on the milk-white beaches and carefully manicured resorts of the larger, more accessible islands like Tahiti, Fiji and Rarotonga. Mangaia, the southernmost of the Cook Islands, was one of the least appealing and most far-flung of all. It had limited fresh water, little electricity, and virtually no tourist trade. The inhabitants dwelt in small poured-concrete huts, living off taro and tinned sardines, and the visitors' accommodation, such as it was, consisted of one boarding house, with a colonial-style bed and a part-time cleaner. Yet although it held little allure for tourists, Mangaia fascinated anthropologists, for since fieldwork had begun in earnest during the late 1960s, its people were said to be special in two distinct respects. First, they held the world record for sexual licentiousness. And second, they had no concept at all of romantic love.

It was these two rumours that Helen Harris had come to investigate, armed with her sixteen-year-old son, a Sony Walkman, and a talent for listening. Harris, the Dean of Students at the University of California in Santa Barbara, was completing her Ph.D. thesis on the nature and evolution of romantic love, and was intrigued by suggestions that right here, in the Pacific Ocean in the twentieth century, there was a culture that had no need for it. No inkling, even, of what it was.

The rumours had started when Donald Marshall, a field anthropologist famous for his work in the South Pacific, paid a visit to Mangaia and fell in with a group of local men. He plied them with beer and asked them to tell him about sexual *mores* on Mangaia. They explained to him in all seriousness that the typical eighteen-year-old Mangaian male experiences three orgasms a night every night of the week, which drops to two orgasms a night five nights a week at the age of twenty-eight, and to one orgasm a night, two to three times a week at the age of forty.

This impressive sexual regime, they maintained, was motivated entirely by pleasure and was completely devoid of the additional complex of emotions that we would characterise as romantic love. Indeed, for both boys and girls, they said, the closest equivalent to the expression 'I love you' could mean only one thing: 'I want to have sex with you.' Marshall's findings were published in 1971 and for a quarter of a century they were accepted without question. But what was the truth? Had he accidentally stumbled on the world's most sex-crazed island, which ignored romantic love in favour of free and frequent congress between both sexes, or was there a different explanation?

It did not take Helen Harris long to find out. Shortly after she arrived on the island, she acquired a small, local-style house and settled in. Her son traded his Walkman for a pig, Helen volunteered to teach some French in the village school, and slowly, both became part of the local community. Gradually at first, and then with increasing frequency, the local people came to tell them their stories.

There was certainly an air of sexual licence about Mangaia. As with many of the Pacific islands, sexual experimentation was considered a natural and inevitable part of growing up. As soon as children reached puberty, they started seeking each other's attentions, at dances, on the road, via sidelong glances in church. However, with a nod to the Christian missionaries who had been busy spreading the Word on the island since the mid-nineteenth century, the actual act of copulation had been driven underground. If individuals wished to have sex, they were obliged to do so covertly, either by absconding into the bushes late at night or, if particularly daring, by having the boy smuggle himself into the girl's house after her parents had gone to sleep. This form of sex, known as *tomo vaine*, or night-crawling, was particularly frowned upon, but it sometimes worked to the boy's advantage, for the punishments which awaited him if he were caught only served to make him appear more daring in the eyes of his beloved.

When Harris asked why night-crawlers were punished, her informants typically reported that it was not because sex as such was wrong, but because the attachments which might be formed could interfere with their parents' carefully laid plans for marriage. Harris was puzzled. Did this mean that some form of romantic love existed on Mangaia? Why, of course, replied the informants. It was one of the major causes of heartache and misery on the island. Why so? Because young people who fell in love didn't think sensibly about whom they should marry. Traditionally, marriage on Mangaia had one primary purpose: to increase the landholdings and prestige of the parents-in-law by having their children joined to rich and successful families. Love, with its apparent whimsicality, paid no attention to sensible considerations like status and wealth, and directed itself often towards the most unsuitable partners. What's more, when lovestruck couples were forced to separate, they pined and complained. Sometimes, they even left the island. And once or twice, suicides had been known. What sort of a feeling was it that caused so much upset, which was so topsy-turvy, which threw reason out of the window and obeyed no laws but its own? What sensible person could understand the point of romantic love, let alone endorse it?

But what about Marshall's claim that the Mangaians knew nothing of love? 'We may not encourage it,' some of the elders replied, 'but that does not mean we know nothing of it.' And their sex-crazed ways? Was it true that the young men had sex two or three times a night every night of the week? 'Where did you hear that?' asked the Mangaians. From Donald Marshall, who visited some years ago. 'Ah, Marshall,' they replied. 'The problem with Marshall was that he believed everything those young boys told him. He'd have got a different story if he'd spoken to the women too. What do you expect if you get a bunch of young men together and get them drunk? They're going to brag about sex!'

When Harris returned to America, after spending a total of nine months on the island, she was a wiser woman. Wherever she had gone, and whoever she had spoken to, everyone knew about love, most had experienced it, and for some (the lucky ones who had fallen for socially advantaged partners) it had even been a factor in marriage. And when she turned her attention away from Mangaia and looked into other cultures, either non-Western where love was said to be absent, or Western cultures from the Classical or pre-modern era, Harris found exactly the same pattern.

From the jungles of the Amazon to the Alaskan Inuit, from the Ifaluk Islanders to the desert nomads, and from ancient Egypt to twentieth-century China, everyone recognised the pangs of romantic love. Everyone was familiar with its joys and agonies, its arbitrary nature, its sudden arrival, and the soul-stripping, heart-swelling, chest-bursting sensations that accompanied its course. But in very few of these places were such emotions considered noble or worthwhile, and almost nowhere were they held to constitute a sensible basis for marriage. The ancient Greeks thought of love as a sort of affliction, like tuberculosis or madness; the Romans considered it a social game; the Japanese relegated it to the role of an enchanting but essentially unreal escape from the deadening routine of duty and family life; and across the world, whatever their opinions about the joy or the worth of love, parents continued to arrange their children's marriages and affairs with ruthless pragmatism.

Perhaps the most illustrative anecdote about attitudes towards love in non-Western cultures was recounted by the doughty anthropologist Dr Audrey Richards, who lived with the Bemba people in what is now Zambia in the 1930s. She recalled that, one evening around the fire, asked to share some of her own folklore, she told a whole village a classic English tale of the exploits of a young prince who climbed mountains, fought monsters, and walked for miles to gain his beloved's hand in marriage and her heart for ever. At the end of her story, she looked around, expecting to see nods of approval and nostalgic smiles. But all she saw was a sea of bewildered, baffled faces, and there was a heavy, awkward silence. Finally, not wishing to seem impolite, but too bewildered to stay quiet any longer, the village head spoke up. 'Why didn't he just find another girl?'

Why, then, have we in the West made such a big deal out of love? Why do we believe that it is the highest expression of our humanity, the end to which we should all strive, the goal, the obligation, often the very purpose of our lives? Why do we want it to be eternal? Why do we run such risks to seek it? And why, of all things, do we marry for it?

Platonic love according to Plato

The story starts in Athens, during the fourth century BC, when the up-and-coming philosopher Plato decides to write a tract entitled *The Symposium*, which celebrates the teachings of his late and great mentor, Socrates. He sets it at the house of Agathon, a tragic poet of the time, and gives it the form of an after-dinner conversation between various Athenian notables, including the comic playwright Aristophanes, the handsome young aristocrat Alcibiades, and, of course, Socrates himself.

The topic under discussion is love: its nature, origin, and purpose. Although Socrates gives the keynote speech, holding that the perfect love is a love of ethereal forms and eternal ideas, it is the playwright Aristophanes' whimsical allegory about love and the origins of humanity which, in the long run, has proved the most enduring.

Aristophanes proposes that once upon a time, when the gods were young and the world was fresh and new, human beings were fashioned from a slightly different mould than the one we know today. Each had four arms, four legs, two faces and a body that could cartwheel at tremendous speeds. The Gods, fearful that these exuberant, athletic beings would soon challenge them for dominion of the Earth, decided to reduce the threat by cutting them all in two. The humans objected but the gods prevailed, and soon each person was sliced perfectly in half, to create two identical forms.

The resulting creatures, the first modern humans, functioned perfectly. They could walk, they could talk, they could laugh, skip, and jump. But deep down inside, turmoil reigned. For each only felt like half a person and desperately wished to be whole again. Some were destined never to find their matching halves, fruitlessly searching year after year, but others were more fortunate. And this, according to Aristophanes, was where love came in, for love was the deep-seated yearning, the desire for total communion, and the strange sense of homecoming which accompanied the meeting of two people who were literally meant for one another. In one of the most expressive passages in all of Plato's writings, Aristophanes describes the feeling:

> No one can suppose that it is mere physical enjoyment which causes one to take such intense delight in the company of the other. It is clear that the soul of each has some other longing which it cannot express but can only surmise and obscurely hint at. Suppose Hephaestus with his tools were to visit them as they lie together, and stand over them and ask: what is it, mortals, that you hope to gain from one another? Suppose too that when they could not answer he repeated his question in these terms: is the object of your desire to be always together as much as possible, and never to be separated from one another day or night? If that is what you want, I am ready to melt and weld you together, so that, instead of two, you shall be one flesh; as long as you live you shall live a common life, and when you die, you shall suffer a common death, and be still one, not two, in the next world. Would such a fate as this content you, and satisfy your longings? We know what their answer would be; no one would refuse the offer; it would be plain that this is what everybody wants, and everybody would regard it as the precise expression of the desire which he had long felt but had been unable to formulate, that he should melt into his beloved, and that henceforth they should be one being instead of two.

This melting, this yearning, this whole-body feeling was exactly what lovers the world over had experienced since the earliest times, but instead of seeing it as an affliction or disease, and instead of imagining it interfered with the proper course of matchmaking, Plato pictured love as an incredibly finely-tuned mechanism which inspired us to seek, recognise and respond to the very person with whom we truly deserved to be joined. Should we somehow fail to seek them or should we find ourselves unwittingly joined to someone else, Plato intimated that we would in some way be failing in our cosmic duty. Should we be energetic enough (or lucky enough) to find them, joys untold would result.

From that moment on, the seeds were sown for a pattern of love that would bear fruit nearly a thousand years later; a pattern which would elaborate on the Greek idea of the search, combine it with a new Christian emphasis on spirituality, add to it a sprinkling of Arab lyricism, and organise them into a structure and format all its own. It would be called courtly love.

Courtly love comes of age

The date: Sunday, 25 April 1227. The place: a road on the Italian mainland near Venice. The occasion: the arrival of the goddess Venus among the ordinary people of Italy. The purpose: to tilt with the knights and squires of the land and win the love of a perfect, unnamed lady.

It was a claim as extravagant as it was extraordinary, and it was the work of a man as typical of his time as he is unusual to ours: the forlorn, lovestruck, seemingly half-crazed Baron Ulrich von Lichtenstein. At any other time or any other place, Ulrich's plan would have had him confined straight to the madhouse. But here, in thirteenth-century Europe, it was a gesture which, though undeniably over the top, by no means condemned him to ridicule. For Ulrich, like many other knights of the time, was seeking a way to express his love for a woman who was, to all intents and purpose, unavailable. She was a Viennese noblewoman of high birth, considerable standing, and an ice-cold, haughty demeanour. He was a younger, lesser figure who, though he had acquired his spurs at the age of twenty-two, could never hope to acquire her. For, added to the social distance between them, she was married. More to the point, so was he.

Nevertheless, this was thirteenth-century Europe, where marriages were brokered not by the individuals concerned but by their parents, and served, among the aristocracy at least, more to cement alliances between families than to indicate affection between individuals. Love could and sometimes did flourish within these bonds, but just as often it did not. And so, to prevent the rebellion of the participants or the social disruption which abandoned marriages might cause, a massive cultural blind eye was turned towards extra-marital desire, a desire which became codified under the system of courtly love.

According to its major principles, perfected at the languorous courts of educated noblewomen like Eleanor of Aquitaine, a knight could, indeed should, declare his love for a well-born lady to whom he was not married. He should go through any number of trials to win her esteem and protect her name. He could then pursue her with all manner of communications and protestations as long as he didn't actually jump into bed with her. It's not clear whether this stipulation was made to guard against the possibility of cuckoldry or whether it arose more in the context of a general, Christian-influenced elevation of the spiritual over the earthly. What is certainly true is that the partial, but not total, reciprocation which courtly love demanded could have been designed as a psychological recipe to maximise fervour.

When Baron von Lichtenstein communicated his interest to his Viennese idol via a song, she behaved in a textbook fashion: distant but not totally dismissive. She told him that he was too lowly for her, that the song was pompous, and that she disliked his harelip. To a less fixated lover, this might have seemed final. But to as dedicated a suitor as Ulrich, it was fuel to the fire. The comment about his lip indicated she had noticed him and surely, if she had noticed him, there was hope. All he had to do was refine his verse, improve his looks, and further his social standing.

His first step was to have the lip surgically repaired, an operation which, given the state of medieval medicine, laid him feverishly in bed for six weeks. His next step was to write a new song, which he duly sent for her approval. And his third step was to start a jousting career which he pursued with such outstanding flair that she could not fail to be impressed. With all these tactics set in motion, Ulrich was once more ready to press his case; he was finally invited to join his lady on a hunting party where, if the occasion arose, he might be permitted to talk to her. Unfortunately, when it did, the knight was so overcome that he found himself unable to utter even a single word. Furious at this display of gaucheness, the lady banished him for ever. Well, not quite for ever. Having seen her at close range, having touched her hand, and having held her attention, if only momentarily, Ulrich was now incapable of turning back.

He fought like never before, underwent numerous adventures and, when he heard that she was displeased with him for falsely boasting he had lost a finger in her service, he promptly hacked it off, encased it in a specially designed velvet pouch, and sent it to her with a lengthy poem about the matter.

Duly impressed, the unnamed lady told Ulrich that she would look at the finger every day, a concession which inspired such a rush of elation that he was led to conceive his ultimate plan, the infamous jousting expedition which would take him from Venice to Vienna, tilting with all the knights of Lombardy, Austria and Bohemia along the way. And just to prove that this expedition was being carried out solely in the name of love, he would attire himself in the garb of the Roman goddess Venus. According to contemporary accounts, the Baron and his retinue made quite a spectacle. The procession was headed by a dozen squires, dressed from head to toe in white. Next came two maids-in-waiting, then a mini-orchestra and, finally, behind them all, a mounted, man-sized figure dressed in an outrageously ornate cream-coloured gown with a heavy veil, a pearl head-dress and waist-length jewel-encrusted braids.

Stopping at frequent intervals to meet his various challengers, Ulrich broke a total of 307 lances. It was a magnificent feat, taking five weeks to accomplish and spreading his name throughout the provinces he visited and even as far as the castle walls of his nameless, faceless lady. When he finally arrived, he was at once given to believe that he would be allowed into her presence, where he could converse and, should he make a sufficiently plausible case, perhaps even kiss her.

In a frenzy of desire, the Baron presented himself at his lady's portals, whereupon he was told to discard his armour and approach her dressed as one of the lepers who habitually begged for alms. Gleefully, the Baron exchanged his finery for rags and bandages and even spent the night in a ditch to add to the air of authenticity. He then threw a rope up to her bedroom window and climbed in to kiss her, only to find that she was surrounded by eight maids-in-waiting, who refused to leave the room. The lady observed Ulrich's frustration, then, while he was still clinging to the rope, took a pair of scissors and cut it from the lintel, sending him hurtling once more down into the moat.

When the Baron looked up again, with an expression not of anger but of sheer, untarnished love, it seems that enough was enough. The game had gone too far, the Baron had proved his constancy and now, finally, he should be granted his reward. And so he was. For instead of sending him away on a crusade, as had originally been planned, the once heartless lady melted into his arms and granted him, after fifteen long years, the delights of her subtle caresses.

What form these caresses took we shall never know, for our information about the Baron is chiefly taken from his own memoirs, related late in life to a scribe and missing in all the intimate details of congress. But if other, similar examples of the culture of courtly love can be used as a guide, he was probably granted the right to remain alone in her company, to kiss her, and possibly to fondle her naked body in bed. Full sexual consummation of their love was not the point and was often not even desired. In those days, knights had prostitutes, serving girls and stable lads to serve their purely sexual impulses.

This was the fulfilment of something different. Something spiritual, something on an altogether different plane. And curiously, as soon as it arrived, it began to wane. For Ulrich, like so many other knights of the period, was no sooner in possession of his prize than he decided to abandon it. Perhaps Ulrich's lady got bored and took another lover, perhaps neither could match up to each other's fantastical expectations, or perhaps, like many a predator and many a prey, they both found that the chase had been more important and more fulfilling than the kill. Either way, the relationship lasted only two years before Ulrich forswore her company for ever and once more took to the road, this time fighting for a different lady, this time dressed as King Arthur of England, and this time even more reckless than before.

What then, has this bizarre institution of courtly love got to tell us? How does it speak to our own generation, nearly one thousand years later, which has long abandoned suits of armour, whose courtships are habitually much more down to earth, and whose marriages, if both parties consent, are usually a matter of individual choice? On one level, the stories of the knights errant are absurd: the indefatigable pursuing the unreachable in search of the unworkable. On the other hand, they served to crystallise a distinct and wholly original view of love; in which the yearning was idealised, the pain transfigured to a sort of latent, slow-burning ecstasy, and the elation transformed from a temporary, transient high to a transcendent, ultimate goal. The core, the essence, the very purpose of life.

Furthermore, the extravagant adventures of the knights errant marked a cultural bridge between the dark ages of barbarism and the new luxuriance of the Renaissance. The courts of Aquitaine might have occupied a different mental universe from the one we live in today, but they helped to usher in a new era of sophistication and literacy which would spread their influence, via the newly invented printing press, to the furthest corners of Europe. Here, generations of readers would indulge their own hunger for similar tales of star-crossed lovers, chivalrous exploits, and ultimate, impossible joy. Lancelot and Guinevere, Tristan and Isolde, and, slightly later, Romeo and Juliet. The great romantic myths of the Western world. Reinvented, elaborated, and dressed in the costumes of each successive age, the power of such tales continues to endure, so that today we are still in thrall to the idea that falling in love is an obligation, the highest ideal, an altar on which all other considerations should be sacrificed. We're in love with love: we adore the idea of its all-consuming power, and wait impatiently to be swept off our feet.

High bridge, low bridge

The Capilano Canyon Suspension bridge is slung across a deep, narrow valley just west of Vancouver. It is five feet wide, four hundred and fifty feet long, and constructed of wooden boards held together by thin wire cables. It dips in the middle, sways in the wind, and shakes with every step you take. To the left and right are breathtaking views of the forests and mountains of the Pacific Northwest. Look down and there is a 230-foot drop to the rocks and rapids below. It's a strange place to study romantic love, but in 1974, for Donald Dutton and Arthur Aron it made perfect sense.

Aron, an erstwhile psychologist with a taste for Eastern mysticism, and Dutton, his more practically minded colleague, had spent many hours discussing the prompts and nudgings of love. Why doesn't it always keep its head down until we meet a suitable partner, lying low through all our fumblings and mistakes and then detonating suddenly when we've finally got it right? We so often seem to fall for people who just aren't right for us, or when we know we aren't in any proper position to get involved, that we can't just be acting out cultural norms or working out sound evolutionary strategies. There must be other factors involved. Factors which make us more vulnerable to falling in love at certain times and not others, almost regardless of whom we meet.

Factors which might depend on our age, our readiness, our mindset, or our mood.

From their perusals of history, philosophy, and the emerging discipline of experimental psychology, Dutton and Aron kept being struck by one common factor: anxiety. Would Romeo and Juliet's love have been so intoxicating had it not been spiced with danger? Would Ulrich's unnamed lady have proved so irresistible had she welcomed him with open arms from the moment they met? And what about Little Green? As she herself may have recognised, there are few things so alluring as the lure of the forbidden. Could it be that an element of high anxiety, whether placed in the lover by their beloved or arising from something beyond either's control, might actually contribute to romantic longing, or even catalyse it?

To try to understand whether this might be the case, Aron spent many weeks combing through the psychological literature. There, he found various studies which claimed to show that susceptibility to romantic attraction increased when people were exposed to threatening, challenging, exertive or exhausting experiences. In other words, experiences which generated high states of physical or psychological arousal. In one study male students who had been viciously berated by their professor were found to have written stories which contained a higher sexual and romantic content than students who had been left alone. In another, women who had been exercising vigorously on a walking machine were found to have reported a greater interest in meeting members of the opposite sex than women who had been sitting still. The evidence was preliminary and poorly focused, but it was a start. It was already a commonplace that people in love felt 'high', – talkative, expansive, more energetic – all characteristic of a state of arousal. Romantic impulses, love, limerence, call it what you will, might, like more general forms of arousal, be most quickly ignited when we find ourselves, through volition or otherwise, in circumstances which produce novel or extreme emotional responses. This then is where the bridge came in.

Together with Dutton, Aron set about trying to devise a situation in which individuals might encounter people about whom they knew very little in circumstances of maximal emotional arousal.

Dutton immediately suggested the bridge, and as soon as Aron made his first journey across, clinging to the handrail, hesitating with each step, and trying not to look at the giddy drop down either side, he was convinced. It was frightening but not too terrifying: people usually undertook the walk for pleasure rather than necessity, as it provided much the same frisson of novelty, exhilaration and terror that generates the peculiar pleasure of horror movies. And as every teenager knows, there is nothing like a late-night horror movie to stimulate seduction.

Best of all, some way downriver there was a much safer bridge: lower, denser, and of more solid construction. This could be used as a control. Here then was the plan. An attractive female confederate would place herself in the middle of each bridge and ask the male bridge-crossers, some of whom had been recruited from Dutton and Aron's university, to fill in a short survey, ostensibly about the effect of scenic views on creative expression. She would then ask them to complete a few details, including age, education, previous visits to the bridge, and so on, and finally, she would ask them to write a short story based around a picture she would have with her. Those who complied would be thanked and sent on their way. But just as they were leaving, the girl would call them back, scribble a telephone number on a piece of paper and tell them that if they wished to know more about the experiment, they were welcome to call her at home.

The day came, the experimenter headed for the bridge, and one by one, men came by and stopped. Meanwhile, back at base, Aron and Dutton were camped by the answer machine. If a call came through for Gloria, they knew they had a high-bridge crosser (for that was the name she had given them). If one came through for Donna, he must be a low-bridger. Slowly, then with increasing frequency, the machine started clicking. 'Hi, Gloria, this is Chuck. We met on the bridge earlier this afternoon. I was wondering if you could give me a call. I'm in psychology too. Here's my number.' 'Gloria, this is Pete. I sure did enjoy the experiment. Please phone me. I'll be in all day.' 'Is that Gloria? Gloria, this is Al. Hi, how are you? I've been thinking about that experiment and I was a little embarrassed about my story. Could you possibly give me a call?' And so it went on. And on. And on. By the end of the day, nine out of a possible eighteen calls had come through for Gloria, while Donna had received only two. What's more, when Aron and Dutton compared the call rate to the amount of sexual imagery in the stories and to the number of men who had agreed to fill in the questionnaires, they found that the high bridge had yielded both a considerably higher acceptance rate and a sexier level of storytelling.

Overall then, what does this experiment have to tell us? That if we're looking to fall in love, we should head for a dangerous bridge, and that if we want our love returned, we should jump on the rails and cross it? Or perhaps, looking at the question from the other way round, that lives in perpetual predictability, without drama or adventure, are doomed to be lived without love? It all seems a bit high-flown and fanciful. Well, yes, but like all figures of speech, especially in the realm of love, it may contain a kernel of truth, revealing something about love's underlying purpose.

Aron, in particular, was so impressed by the results of this experiment that he's gone on investigating love ever since. These days, he's a little wry about the bridge study. 'We were all pretty young,' he says, 'and we weren't really into sexual equality in those days.' But nevertheless, it proved an important step in developing the theory he holds to now: that romantic love has been designed as a vital tool to expand the self. According to this theory, love is the most effective means of motivating individuals to expand and take another person into their lives. By blending and melding with them, they can then gain and enjoy each other's perspectives, resources and so forth and, metaphorically speaking, have use of everything in the other's house as well as in one's own. It was Platonic philosophy and evolutionary theory all in one and, to test it, Aron devised two simple experiments.

In the first, he asked 325 undergraduate students to complete a questionnaire once a fortnight over a ten-week period which simply asked them what sort of person they were and whether they had fallen in love over the last two weeks. When people had not fallen in love, their descriptions of themselves were short and unvarying but when they had, these grew considerably in both length and breadth. The second experiment was more subtle. Here, people in long-term relationships were given a long list of adjectives and asked to tell the experimenter whether they applied to themselves, their partner, both, or neither. A short while later they were presented with the same list again, and asked whether the adjectives were true just of themselves. In nearly all cases, the fastest responses were given to those adjectives that were true of both the individuals and their partners, and the slowest responses to those which were simply true of themselves. This seemed to indicate that the individuals had merged with their partners to such an extent that they had to mentally reverse themselves out of the relationship before being able to think about themselves in isolation.

By considering these experiments in tandem, and also by dwelling a little on the lexicon of love ('I'm bursting with happiness', 'We melted into each other's arms', 'I was lost in his gaze' and so on), Aron, now working with his wife Elaine, perceived that there did indeed seem to be a sense in which lovers were melded, fused, joined at the hip. And that the resulting whole seemed to be larger and more effective than the sum of its parts.

Thus, the high bridge suggests, however metaphorically, that those who dare not expand, either because they're struggling to keep pace with the lives they've already got, or because they're frightened of the unknown, the potential loss of control, the giddying heights and hurtling lows of uncertainty, may close a protective carapace over their lives which forbids entry from the outside. In some cases, this may be a lifelong condition, resulting from the sort of attachment disorders identified in the last chapter, but for some it may be a temporary state, brought on by an impossibly heavy workload, a sudden lack of self-confidence, or a stony self-reliance. These types wouldn't ever have got on to the high bridge in the first place.

On the other hand, for those who are open to love – open to life – the bridge experiment might strike a chord. The newspapers are full of stories of holiday romances, catalysed by the lure of the exotic, the thrill of the unfamiliar, the promise of something different and dangerous. Such liaisons may not often last. For a start, they often lack the components of similarity and complementarity which contribute to the full experience of love, but that's not what Aron's work is about. It concerns what sparks off love, not what makes it endure. And just as mildly pleasant anxiety-producing states can help to generate it, so can unpleasant ones. The phenomenon of wartime romance is the stuff of fact as well as fiction, brought on and souped up by the wail of air-raid sirens, the close huddles in the underground shelters, and the whistling of bullets and bombs. Would *Gone With the Wind* have been so romantic had it not been set against the flaming backdrop of the Civil War? And just why do so many soldiers feel the need to write and receive romantic letters, even from total strangers, during times of stress and conflict?

In more mundane circumstances, the same phenomenon can sometimes be observed in people who have been trapped in a lift together, who are joined by a common difficulty, or who have undertaken an arduous journey in each other's company. Art Aron was even able to create the first stirrings of romantic love in a laboratory, by taking two complete strangers and locking them in a room together for an hour and a half, where each was obliged to ask the other a series of increasingly intimate questions. At the end of the session, most reported strong feelings of romantic attraction which equalled or even outweighed those they felt towards their long-term partner. (Aron remembers more than one worried partner pacing the halls outside his lab while their beloved shared intimate information with a stranger.) The feelings induced this way don't always last, but sometimes they do. The first pair he experimented on even ended up getting married, with Aron and his team as guests of honour at the wedding.

Seen from the high bridge, Ulrich von Lichtenstein's antics no longer seem so utterly alien to us. If well-nourished, sensible Canadian psychology students in the twentieth century can be nudged into romantic action by just crossing a bridge, perhaps it's not so ludicrous that a hungry, fanatical, repressed medieval knight would be willing to risk death just for a kindly word from his beloved. People all over the world, and throughout history, have fallen in love despite the risks, quite possibly because above all else, the sheer rush of it felt so good. But our cultural inheritance of courtly love, and the belief in love as an all-conquering force, cuts both ways. Happily perhaps, we are now encouraged to direct it towards more realistic partners. Less happily, many feel that they have failed when the love they experience is less than all-consuming or permanently enduring.

Love that lasts

Kerstin Uvnas-Moberg is a researcher at the Karolinska Institute in Stockholm who believes that our inherited idea of love is simply missing the point. Or rather, that it only provides half the picture. If there were nothing more to love than the sort of revved-up, hyperactive, desperate, sleepless yearning that characterised Ulrich's feelings toward his beloved, Romeo's towards Juliet, or Isolde's towards Tristan, love would be a strange beast indeed. Unwieldy, unhelpful; in fact, evolutionarily unsound. It would lead us into one risky situation after another, so hooked on excitement we'd never be able to settle down long enough to make sure our genes prospered. We need a degree of energy to pursue our loved ones, to be sure, and we need the resilience and motivation to conquer initial rejection, or we might never have a chance of winning anyone, yet the quelling of such all-consuming passion and the subsidence of the full-blown state of limerence is essential if we are to be led into the sort of enduring and mutually satisfying relationships that love as a whole was originally designed to promote.

Uvnas-Moberg, whose garrulous manner and infectious giggle belie a profoundly serious intent, is one of the world's leading researchers into a hormone called oxytocin. Secreted deep inside the hypothalamus and regulated by the brain's master switch, the pituitary gland, oxytocin may be partly responsible for weaning us off the initial, exhilarating souped-up state of romance and for starting to convert it to something quite different, a state of calm and quiet joy.

The influence of chemicals like oxytocin on our behaviour is one of the most complex and fascinating areas in all biology, and it's one where there's still a great deal more to find out. Again and again, research shows tentative links between specific chemicals, and almost as soon as the findings are published, it emerges that the original chemical is actually a compound of several separate and independent substances, which subtly shift their balance and overall level in a constant response to conditions outside the body. The sheer number of hormones, and their sometimes contradictory effects, means that endocrinologists have their work cut out just keeping up with the trade literature. Yet this is the field where drug companies will probably make much of their money during the next century. Best-selling pills like Prozac, fast-acting detox treatments for drug addicts and maybe even improved medication for schizophrenia all depend on a better understanding of the literally mind-boggling mixture of chemicals in our heads.

There are four fundamental families of neurochemicals – substances released within the brain, in both men and women – which make us feel good and fluctuate according to our circumstances. Like the testosterone and oestrogen we've met in previous chapters, they are hormones, but unlike them they're more subtle and elusive, they're headquartered in the brain, and their effects are much more similar in both sexes. The best-known is adrenaline, that kick-start to the system which is probably one of the major players in our initial exhilaration in love. But it's also the footsoldier of our body's primal 'fight or flight' response, triggered in response to threatening situations and preparing us for immediate action. Blood is diverted to the muscles, the heart pumps faster, sugar levels rise At the same time, the digestive system closes down, the mouth dries and whatever nutrients are lurking in the stomach cease to be absorbed. The mental state is one of hyper-awareness, of absolute preparedness. Both body and mind are ready for action.

Like the other neurochemicals, adrenaline has to be balanced out in incredibly fine quantities to work properly. Our brains also respond to our circumstances with a delicate mix of other neurochemicals, chief among them dopamine, serotonin and endorphins. These have an equally radical effect on the way we feel. Then, swirling around in this heady brew, there are two additional and somewhat mysterious substances which have been implicated in our behaviour in love. First there's phenylethlamine, more handily known as PEA, which seems to be one of the chemicals which gives us that 'walking on air' feeling familiar to anyone who's been impulsively and suddenly in love. It's even been suggested – probably inaccurately – that PEA is 'the romance hormone', and serial fallers-in-love have chronically low PEA levels which they seek to boost with continuous romantic intrigues.

Finally, there's Uvnas-Moberg's favourite chemical: oxytocin. For many years oxytocin has been known as the hormone associated with child-birth, bringing on strong contractions in labour and cutting down on post-partum bleeding. But Uvnas-Moberg is now showing that oxytocin has a far wider armoury of powers, and that its effects may not be just physical but psychological as well.

Uvnas-Moberg, like the attachment theorists we met in the last chapter, is fascinated by the interaction between mother and baby. She, too, wants to know why some mothers seem to bond so quickly and thoroughly with their babies, while others never quite get the hang of it. But rather than simply observing their behaviour, she wants to get right inside their bodies, measuring and analysing the invisible but overwhelming tides of oxtytocin in the mothers' bloodstreams. And in the cosy, comfortable rooms where the Karolinska Institute places new mothers and their babies, she's been doing just that. It's a great place to work: although the babies occasionally grizzle and squall, the overall atmosphere is one of extraordinary calm and contentment. Nobody here ever seems to be pitched into a fight-or-flight pattern. Instead, as the mothers concentrate on breastfeeding their newborns, the rooms are suffused with a hazy warmth, inwardly reflective, almost sluggish. And as Uvnas-Moberg takes blood samples and analyses their content, she finds an interesting pattern. Mothers with the highest oxytocin levels are not just producing the most milk, they're also feeling the most satisfied, encouraged into the sort of relaxed, sedate state of mind essential for both mother and baby to get properly attached to each other.

It might seem a classic example of the feedback loops which plague investigation into hormones, a chicken-and-egg situation where one can't pick out what comes first – the hormone, the behaviour it encourages but which, in turn, raises its levels, or the psychological state which motivates the behaviour. Disentangling cause and effect was going to be a puzzle, but with oxytocin it seemed particularly important, for if a hormone had such significant effects on our earliest and deepest experiences of love, it might well have more to tell us about love in later life.

And soon, Uvnas-Moberg found that it probably did, for oxytocin is naturally produced not just during the critical periods surrounding birth and during breastfeeding, but also in response to three further activities: stroking, kissing and lovemaking. Furthermore, this effect was not just confined to women. A few years ago, tests conducted on masturbating males showed that it spiked at the very moment of ejaculation, possibly contributing to the pleasure of orgasm and certainly to the feeling of happy lassitude which followed. And just recently, Uvnas-Moberg has also found that slow but steady increases also occur during massage. In one instance, after a particularly lengthy and relaxing session, one man showed oxytocin levels which equalled even those of a nursing mother. These mutually shared episodes of kissing, touching and fondling, which were for Ulrich the end of the line, are for many of us just the beginning.

So it seems that love may come in two distinct packages, each with its own complement of neurochemicals and its own specific function. First there's an initial rush of energy and exhilaration generated by adrenaline and related substances, which is designed to make us overcome the obstacles between ourselves and our loved one. Then, there's a second, calmer, more pleasurable state associated with oxytocin, which helps to foster the sort of stable, long-term relationship that would lead to the generation and protection of our progeny.

True love, then, as every wise old adviser knows, is more than the state of limerence. More than the crazy feeling which had Ulrich by the throat, Romeo and Juliet on their knees, and poor old Dr Vesteroy in despair. It shifts from peaks and troughs of romantic longing to the verdant pastures of going steady. From the thrill of the chase to the more recumbent pleasures of permanence and parenthood. From the joy of the proposal to the calm mundanity of marriage. And just as our love shifts, we shift too. We regain our appetites, catch up on lost sleep, and exchange our stockings and stilettos for warm, cosy slippers and long evenings in. Once slaves to our emotions, we become, at least partially, their masters, and from being deeply *in* love with our partners, we come to love them deeply.

But if this, from a biochemical point of view, accounts for the whys, whens and wherefores of romantic love, what about that crucial ingredient, the indispensable who? Are there really particular people with whom we're destined to fall in love? If so, how can we be sure we've found them?

Perfect love takes a fall

Justin and Ursula met in the summer of 1964. He was a sixteen-year-old British public schoolboy with wealthy, well-connected parents and a bright future ahead of him. She was a Hungarian émigré who had escaped across the Austrian border with a sheepskin coat, snowboots, a pocketful of food and little else. She was also more than ten years his senior. They had met one evening when she was visiting his parents with her husband. For Justin, it was love at first sight. That night, he crept up to her bedroom and deposited a note under her door telling her he loved her. The next day, she disappeared. The following summer, when he was seventeen, Justin drove down to the South of France, where his parents had rented a villa. There she was once again, sitting in the garden on a swing seat. He was just as smitten. He walked straight up to her and told her again that he loved her. She burst into tears. A few weeks later, she decided to leave her husband and spend the rest of her life with Justin. For the next seventeen years, they travelled all over the world, with no one but each other for company. They became obsessed with each other. They couldn't leave each other's sight. Their passion was so all-consuming that not even Justin's family could come near them. As Justin's brother, Tim, wrote in his subsequent book about their relationship, *The Monument*, their passion was such that there was no room for close friends, confidants, even brothers.

Then, one day late in 1981, after nearly two decades during which they had come to complement each other 'like fruit perfectly joined from two component halves', Ursula was suddenly found dead in her hotel room with a revolver and a stack of sleeping pills by her side. From the documents around her, including her diary, it seemed that she could not bear the thought of growing old. At the age of forty-four, she had just begun to feel the first inklings of mortality, and her love had hitherto been so passionate, so dedicated, so all-consuming that the idea that it might be starting to wane had filled her with a dread more terrible than death. When Justin heard the news, he was inconsolable. He haunted the places they had once visited, returned home to be with his parents, then stalked the streets of London looking for something, anything that reminded him of her. A few months later, he returned to Africa, where they had spent so much time together, and shot himself through the head. Tim went out to fetch the body, which had been discovered in a Khartoum hotel room surrounded by pictures of Ursula, and took it to nearby Nyala, where he knew Justin wished to be buried. Here, he found Ursula's grave, with a space beside it and an inscription in Greek, which read 'Ursula and Justin – One'. His place was already waiting.

On one level, Ursula and Justin's story is the pinnacle of the Western romantic ideal, combining Plato's idea of two predestined souls with the courtly components of danger, passion and doom. However, rather than bemoan the fact that such heights of adoration and such perfect, soul-drenching unions are not the legitimate inheritance of every lover, we should give thanks for their very rarity.

If love really were to function like that, with a single perfect partner for every person alive, with thunderclaps if we found them and disappointment if we didn't, our race could never have survived. Bearing in mind that the global population currently stands at nearly six billion people, the odds of finding our single perfect soulmate would be small indeed, and even if we succeeded, the sudden burst of fireworks which followed might make the lifelong association designed to ensue seem a very poor second. This was exactly the problem with Ursula, who was unable to cope when the liquid passion which had soldered her to Justin finally began to cool and crack.

Happily, when one considers love's design, it is a little more forgiving and a little more elastic. For love has developed in the human psyche not to help us find *the* perfect partner but to help us find *a* suitable partner at *the* right time. And suitability, rather than perfection, is the key. Consider what makes us attracted to some people and not to others. In the last chapter, I suggested that two sorts of forces were at work. First, universal signals of youth, health, and fertility, the worldwide indicators of beauty. Second, a set of individual characteristics which play into the knots and grooves of our own childhoods and upbringing. Perfection blended with particularity. Now let me introduce a third component, a component which separates those with whom we may fall in love from those whom we simply sexually desire. This third component we might term complementarity.

Similar but different

Of the following two statements, which is the more true? First: opposites attract. Second: like attracts like. In the realm of human relations, the question has been much debated. Various studies during the 1960s and early 1970s, notably those by Elaine and G. William Walster, suggested the former. When individuals were asked to choose between several types of people, all of whom were very attracted to them, they tended to choose those who were most dissimilar. With an eye to the Western heritage of doomed love, this was promptly christened the Romeo and Juliet effect. However, at just about the same time, an equally large body of work, chiefly conducted by Donn Byrne and his colleagues, appeared to show quite the opposite. In his experiments, people seemed to express a clear preference for those who were very similar to them, in both looks and personality. This we might term the Narcissus effect, after the character from Greek mythology who fell in love with his own reflection.

In more recent times, intriguing support for the Narcissus effect has been found by David Perrett, a psychologist at the University of St Andrews who studies components of sexual attractiveness. Like Judith Langlois and Victor Johnston from the last chapter, Perrett creates computer-generated images of individual faces, averaged faces, and ideal faces, and asks subjects to rate them. Like Langlois, he finds that average faces are rated higher than individual faces, and like Johnston, he finds that ideal faces are rated higher still. But Perrett also goes one step further. With a highly sophisticated morphing programme and acting on a hunch all his own, he then photographs the face of the actual rater, subtly changes its sex, then feeds that into the computer as well. As a result, males are looking at female versions of themselves, and females at male versions. When asked to rate these alongside the individual faces, the average faces and the ideal faces, many of them rate the sex-changed version of their own face, which they never recognise as their own, as the most attractive of all. There is something ineffable to it, something which almost beckons them in.

On the surface, this seems a little surprising. Quasimodo would still look like Quasimodo whatever sex you made him, and surely he would still prefer Esmerelda. What's more, as we've seen from studies into smell and theories about the basic rationale for sexual reproduction, surely it would make the most sense to go for people who are different from us, for different looks indicate different genes, and different genes make for better, more robust children.

Well yes, but think again. Many of us may sexually desire women who look like Marilyn Monroe or men with the charisma and influence of JFK, but most of us don't fall in love with them because there's so little chance that they will love us back. So here's love's secret safety-catch. It's not a simple, one-sided emotion which we foist full-blown on whomever we desire in the hope that they will magically return it. In our own day, such one-sided love affairs have resulted in the phenomenon of celebrity-stalking, whose most extreme expression is De Clérambault syndrome, where the lover deludes himself into believing that the man or woman he worships might somehow love him back. The first recorded case was of a woman who stood outside the gates of Buckingham Palace every day, firm in the belief that she was having a passionate affair with George V. Such emotions are fine as teenage fads or passing fantasies, but they don't help at all in the real world of adult relationships, where reciprocation is the necessary precursor to our species' underlying purpose: reproduction.

Far from picking on those who will never give us the time of day, romantic love has developed to lead us into mutually satisfying and durable relationships, the sort of relationships needed to raise a family and give our genes the best chance in future generations. As a result, it would make sense if love were to balance the recognition of perfection with the probability of reciprocation, and to hold back from detonating fully unless reciprocation were in the air. And, according to Donn Byrne, Art Aron and others who have studied the subject, one of the most reliable guides to reciprocation is the degree of similarity. Those who are similar to us in looks, skills and personality are more likely to love us back than those who are way out of our league.

Evolutionary psychologist Bruce Ellis has an interesting way of communicating this to his students. He takes a group of thirty and sticks a numbered card on each of their foreheads. The students are then asked to pair up with the highest rating number they can. Naturally, everyone starts to cluster around number thirty, but number thirty is not interested in anyone except number twenty-nine. As a result, these two pair up and leave the rest to cluster around number twenty-eight. The whole charade starts again until eventually, number twenty-eight is paired with number twenty-seven, number twenty-six with number twenty-five, and so on right down the line.

Just as in Ellis's experiment, so in real life. Unable to interest those with the highest mate value, unless we're irresistible ourselves, most people have to adjust their sights downwards until they settle on a partner who is likely to accept them. Although every potential partner will have a different mix of advantages to offer, nine times out of ten, the eventual match will be someone who has an overall mate value very similar to their own.

This then may be the very reason why, as Tennov and Stendhal noticed, lovers have a tendency to exaggerate the positive qualities of their loved ones and either ignore or relish their negative ones. In Stendhal's terms, we may fall in love with a stick but it helps if we perceive it as a diamond wand. In Ellis's, we may be obliged to settle for a five, but it helps if we perceive it as a ten. The blindness of love so often remarked on by poets and philosophers has not evolved as a cruel and random trick but specifically in order to reconcile us to the types of partner we have a chance of winning – and keeping.

This explains perfectly why, although we desire perfection, we fall in love with people who are broadly similar to ourselves. Within these ground rules, it also accounts for the apparently contradictory results obtained by the Walsters. Here, if you remember, subjects were asked to choose between a range of different partners, all of whom were very attracted to them. When they did so, they passed over the very similar partners in favour of others who were completely different. Fine. But remember, these people already had the assurance that all the partners were interested in them. With the knowledge that they were not going to be wasting their time chasing after people who might never reciprocate, their similarity detectors had seized up and been replaced by what might be called complementarity detectors – detectors which zeroed in on the best and most varied balance of qualities which could be exchanged and interwoven with their own. The best and most perfect matches of all, generally speaking, are therefore those where mutual attraction is teamed with complementarity. He's good at some things, she's good at others. He's creative, she's practical. He's a great cook, she's good at languages. He's an occasional genius, she's a better communicator. In this way, rather than doubling up and competing at the same narrow range of skills, a greater range of tasks can successfully be accomplished, and a greater range of qualities (not to mention a more varied set of genes) passed down from parents to child.

So, returning to the original question, whether opposites attract or like attracts like, the frustrating yet inevitable answer is that both do. In ideal circumstances, we fall in love with people who are broadly similar to ourselves, yet different enough to make the result of our union add up to more than the sum of its parts. Yet, as we've seen throughout this book, the idea of one man and one woman living together in perfect harmony, content with each other and only each other from the moment they meet until their dying day, is more often than not an unrealistic ambition.

Love and marriage

What then is the true nature of the long-term relationship between love and marriage? Can they really go together like the proverbial horse and carriage, or are the stresses and strains of a life lived juggling the demands of children, house, work and spouse almost guaranteed to destroy it? And if love does flounder, what should we do? Rush about trying to plug the leaks and bale out our vessels, hoping against hope that we will drift back out into the open seas and clear blue skies of our once-perfect union? Accept that every boat leaks and simply be content to paddle along, keeping our heads more or less above water most of the time? Or should we rather, at the first sign of trouble, run for the gunwales, abandon ship, and immediately look to board a smarter, newer vessel?

Anthropologist Helen Fisher firmly believes the latter. Moreover, she thinks that divorce and the death of love might have been a problem since the very earliest times. In poring over the United Nations divorce statistics for sixty-two peoples around the world, she noticed that a vastly disproportionate number occurred after approximately four years of marriage, exactly the sort of period when any initial love bond was likely to have diminished and not yet been replaced by the full complement of long-term chemicals (or long-term attachment, if you prefer a psychological explanation). Fisher's interest in evolution meant that it didn't surprise her at all to discover that the most common causes of divorce, all around the world, were infidelity and infertility. That much was straightforward. If one's chances of passing on one's genes are frustrated by a sterile or cheating partner, better by far to give up.

But Fisher took the logic even further. The overwhelming peak of divorce after three or four years of marriage, she believes, is really evolution's way of telling us that, having paired up for long enough to conceive and rear one child, we should be looking out to pair with someone else and conceive another, creating an ever more varied genetic legacy. However, the study has several flaws. First, falling in love exacts considerable costs in terms of time and energy. Why do it more often than you have to? Second, flying the marital nest will mean some period, at least, on one's own. Why take the risk? And third, how sure can we be that the next spouse will be better than the last – or kinder to a child who is not even their own? Surely, unless we know we're on to a permanent loser, it's better to try to stick with the partner we've got rather than re-enter the lottery time after time.

Art Aron, who has studied marriages right over the life course, agrees with Fisher that the early years can be very difficult, but suggests that different forces are at work. He attributes the strain some couples feel not to the desire for genetic variety but to the loss of opportunities for expansion. In the early, heady years of a relationship, as the couple find out new things about each other, share new experiences, and undertake the task of moving in together, getting married, and starting a family, they are constantly expanding and fusing. However, as life becomes increasingly routine and each individual gets to know the nooks and crannies of the other's personality, tastes, memories and experiences, opportunities for further expansion diminish. This, he suggests, is a natural part of the human condition, and rather than try to jump ship, we should undertake relationship-building tasks together: holiday versions of the high bridge experiment, like skydiving or bungee-jumping, or taking each other on exotic holidays. Anything that is likely to recapture the feelings of elation, novelty, and pleasurable anxiety which characterised our early years.

Perhaps the most useful studies on what will split and what will bond a couple have been made by John Gottman in Seattle, a kindly psychologist whose offices overlook Lake Washington, out towards the distant horizons of the Pacific, towards Hawaii, towards Mangaia, and towards Pitcairn, where we began this story.

Gottman operates the largest love and marriage lab in the United States, designed to monitor the nature and progress of the typical modern marriage. Here, couples whose relationships are notably good or notably bad, and some whose relationships are just average, come to be scrutinised by Gottman and his ten-strong team. First, they spend twenty-four hours in his experimental apartment, a living space in which the couples pass what they consider to be a typical day. With cameras on the walls, microphones in the living room, and test tubes in the bathroom which collect spittle and urine samples, Gottman analyses every detail of their actions and interactions, looking for points of stress, marks of affection, arguments and their resolutions.

After that, both members of the couple enter Gottman's office and talk through their relationship as they see it. They describe how they met, what attracted them to each other, when they got married, who made what arrangements, and how they have found living together and bringing up their children. They introduce some of the conflicts that typically occur, and try to describe how they resolve them. From this interview alone, Gottman claims to be able to predict with 94 per cent accuracy whether couples will stay together or whether they are bound for the rocky road towards dissolution or divorce. But the real fun starts later, when the couple are taken to his hi-tech lab and sat down, strapped in and wired up to a vast array of technological equipment. With EKG electrodes taped to their chests, sweat and heart-rate detectors on their fingertips, breathing-rate bands around their diaphragms, and a camcorder inches from their faces, Gottman then asks them to discuss an area of continuing conflict in their relationship.

The same themes crop up over and over again. He doesn't talk, she doesn't listen; the kids are destroying their sex lives; their days are so ordinary, so boring; they never have time for each other; they don't share any interests; their love has lost its sparkle; their lives have gone stale. However, the difference between this discussion and the normal, everyday marital moaning sessions that can be heard up and down the country, across the seas and all over the world is that here, every breath, every heartbeat, every rise and fall of the voice, every twitch of the hands and every tiny shuffle of the feet is being monitored, measured, scanned and compared by a team of highly trained relationship technicians. And at their head, presiding over the murky waters of marriage like a modern-day Neptune, is the grey-bearded, twinkly-eyed Gottman.

'It's an amazing experience,' he reports, 'like seeing a CAT scan of a living relationship.' However, unlike a CAT scan, the read-out doesn't relate to the linear reasoning of the brain, but to the elusive, constantly shifting tides of the heart. 'I feel like a fifteenth-century Portuguese explorer,' he reflects. 'We have maps, but not very good ones. I'm trying to chart new territory. To make a map of the human heart.' But what, from all the read-outs, print-outs, monitors and microphones, has he discovered?

The most important thing of all, Gottman suggests, is not how much the couple argues, how many problems each partner has with the other (you inherit a set of unchangeable problems whoever you're with), or even how much each is tempted to stray. Rather, it is in the way the couple *deals* with conflicts and problems when they do arise. Some argue a lot but find that the thrill of making up more than compensates for the cost of the conflict; some argue very little, preferring to skim over disagreements and concentrate on the positive side of their relationship, and some spend so much time compromising that disagreements rarely occur.

All these patterns are common and all are reliably healthy. But there is one category of behaviours which, if he perceives them, Gottman knows may ruin an otherwise stable marriage. So destructive are these behaviours that he labels them 'the four horsemen of the apocalypse'. They are *criticism* (attacking a partner's personality or behaviour); *contempt* (sneering or scoffing at one's partner); *defensiveness* (denying responsibility for a problem and blaming one's partner instead); and *stonewalling* (withdrawing from an argument and facing one's partner with a stony silence and a refusal to re-engage). Everyone displays one or more of these behaviours from time to time, but the persistent, unmitigated employment of such techniques, especially if unmodified by moments of support, love, and mutual affection, is a sure-fire sign of imminent crisis and ultimate collapse.

Not only that: according to Gottman they can be as dangerous to our physical health as they are to our psychological well-being. In one study, Gottman and his team found that the level of criticism and contempt displayed by a couple towards each other bore a direct relation to the number of infectious diseases from which they would suffer over the next five years. The higher the level of criticism, the more prevalent and virulent the infections. The reason for this, explains Gottman, is that when both partners in a couple behave negatively towards one another, particularly when they display one of the 'four horsemen', their blood pressure rises, their stress levels increase, and their excitatory systems start working overtime, making them feel restless and potentially aggressive.

In the early stages of a relationship, when both parties are seeking to win each other over and are blind to each other's faults, stress and excitation can be pushed in a positive direction and interpreted as a pleasant state – even when they arise from a squabble or a row. Once they've been together for several years, however, and the initial sheen of infatuation has dulled under life's demands, marriage should come to function like a port in a storm of life, and not like another storm. We just don't have the energy to cope with continual problems at home as well as in the outside world. We want peace, comfort, and security, both as giver and receiver. This is why, as couples all over the world have discovered, the reintroduction of excitatory hormones does not tend to kick-start their relationship, but to kick it in the teeth. It is also why, rather than struggling to make themselves more attractive to their once idealised partners, the disillusioned often react with anger and derision, and see each other's faults more clearly than ever before.

In marriages where the four horsemen keep rearing their heads, indeed in all marriages, Gottman's sage and simple advice is to make room for the other person, to try to soothe them and, if you really can't avoid occasionally criticising your partner, at least to make sure you mitigate that criticism with a much higher ratio of praise, encouragement and support. Like all good advice, it makes sense on paper but is cripplingly hard to put into practice. Why, then, do we have so much difficulty in keeping love alive for long?

It may be that regardless of love's function in furthering our genetic interests, we simply haven't evolved to love in the way we feel we should – faithfully, fondly and for ever. In today's world, our marriages are under far greater stress than at any other time in human history. Most obviously, we live for a great deal longer, putting demands on our relationship which most of our ancestors would never have had to bear. We're surrounded by cultural messages urging individual fulfilment at the expense of all else.

More and more, as people's links to their families, their place of birth, and their work are considered temporary and replaceable, we put all our emotional eggs into one basket, that of a solid, yet passionate romantic relationship. And unlike the vast majority of humans before us, we now place romantic love at the very heart of marriage, expecting it to last without dying away or even changing much, however much we age and change ourselves. As if this ever-growing burden of expectation weren't enough, separation for the disillusioned is now perhaps easier than it's ever been before. Small wonder that 50 per cent of all new marriages now end in divorce.

Yet despite this combination of trials, and despite the numerous alternative ways of arranging human sexual relations, from the free-for-alls on Pitcairn to the free love of the Oneidans, from the polygamy of the Hebrew patriarchs to the celibacy of the early Christians, from the harem-building early emperors to the half-crazed thirteenth-century courtly lovers, the union of one man and one woman, for better or worse, for richer for poorer, till death do them part, is still as sensible and realistic a way of trying to optimise human relations and contribute to the greater happiness, peace and stability of mankind as any of the myriad alternatives. That's not to say it's foolproof, nor that it is the right method for every man and woman alive. But the fact that 50 per cent of marriages fail means that 50 per cent also endure. And in a species which emerges with the scars and trophies resulting from three and a half billion years of lying, cheating, bullying and manipulation, this is cause for celebration and, perhaps, for hope.

To the reader

If you feel your own experiences would help to elucidate some of the themes in this book, the author would be pleased to hear from you. Please write to PO Box 4765, London SE11 1XA, or e-mail:

anatomy.desire@optomen.co.uk

Acknowledgements

During the time I've been writing and producing programmes about sexuality, I've had the privilege of meeting and corresponding with many of the most illustrious names in sex research. My thanks go to John Bancroft and John Money in particular, who have been a personal as well as a professional inspiration, but also to everyone else who has allowed me or my colleagues to pick their brains and whose work is reflected, directly or indirectly, in this book. They include Gene Abel, Henry Adams, Laura Allen, Deb Alley, Art Aron, Michael Bailey, Robin Baker, Gregory Ball, Howard Barbaree, David Barlow, Judith Becker, Mark Bellis, Fred Berlin, Mitch Berman, Laura Betzig, Monique Borgerhoff Mulder, Donald Brown, Vern Bullough, David Buss, Bram Buunk, Donn Byrne, Sybil Carrere, Sue Carter, Elizabeth Cashdan, Russell Clark, Peggy Cohen-Kettenis, Eli Coleman, Leda Cosmides, Theresa Crenshaw, David Crews, Tim Crow, Antonio Damasio, Martin Daly, Richard Davenport-Hines, Mildred Dickemann, Park Dietz, Russell and Rebecca Dobash, Robin Dunbar, Don Dutton, Bruce Ellis, Nancy Etcoff, Peter Fenwick, Helen Fisher, Michael Gazzaniga, Jay Giedd, Brian Gladue, Raymond Goodman, Guy Goodwin, Louis Gooren, Roger Gorski, John Gottman, Charlotte Graham, Karl Grammer, Richard Green, David Greenberg, Edgar Gregersen, Tom Gregor, Dean Hamer, William Hamilton, Helen Harris, Elaine Hatfield, Kristen Hawkes, Cindy Hazan, Julia Heiman, Gilbert Herdt, Eric Hickey, Elizabeth Hill, Stephen Hucker, Elaine Hull, Sarah Hrdy, Tom Insel, William Jankowiak, Phillip Jenkins, Victor Johnston, Steve Jones, Harold Jordan, Astrid Jütte, Nancy Kalish, Louise Kaplan, Jonathan Ned Katz, Douglas Kenrick, Chris Knight, Ellen Laan, Ron Langevin, Thore Langfeldt, Judy Langlois, Joseph LeDoux, Harold Leitenberg, Simon

LeVay, Robert Levenson, Roy Levin, Elliott Leyton, Hanny Lightfoot-Klein, Stafford Lightman, Roland Littlewood, David Lykken, Neil Malamuth, William Marshall, John Manning, John Maynard Smith, Cindy Meston, Geoffrey Miller, Steven Mithen, David Nias, Tuppy Owens, Constance Penley, James R. Pennebaker, Derek Perkins, David Perrett, Bruce Perry, Jonathan Pincus, Roy Porter, Nick Pound, Camilla Power, Vern Quinsey, Russell Reid, Robert Ressler, Anja Rikowski, Lori Roggman, Duncan Rowland, David Rubinow, Hector Sabelli, Peter Salovey, David Scharff, Joanna Scheib, Greg Simpson, Dev Singh, Koos Slob, Robert C. Solomon, Lawrence Stone, Dick Swaab, Donald Symons, Reay Tannahill, Tim Taylor, Dorothy Tennov, Randy Thornhill, Lionel Tiger, John Tooby, Maryon Tysoe, Kerstin Uvnas-Moberg, Sanderijn van der Doef, Kim Wallen, Harry Walsh, Ian Watts, Claus Wedekind, Jeffrey Weeks, Jim Weinrich, Estela Welldon, Aron and Leonard Weller, Beverley Whipple, Greg White, Michael Wiederman, George Williams, Edward O. Wilson, Glenn Wilson, Margo Wilson and Michael Zona.

I'd also like to thank those who have shared their personal stories, many of them for the first time. While the majority of these have not been included in this book, a small number have. Therefore, my special thanks go to Terri and Kim, Gary and Peter, Ray Tyles, Nelson Cooper, Mark Matthews, and Karen Greenlee.

Bibliography

Abel, G. G., Becker, J. V., Cunningham-Rathner, J., Mittelman, S., and Rouleau, J.-L., 'Multiple Paraphilic Diagnoses Among Sex Offenders', *Bulletin of the American Academy of Psychiatry and the Law*, 16:2, 153–68

Abel, G. G., and Blanchard, E. B., 'The Role of Fantasy in the Treatment of Sexual Deviation', *Archives of General Psychiatry*, 30, 467–75, 1974

Abel, G. G., Mittelman, M. S., and Becker, J. V., 'Sex Offenders: Results of Assessment and Recommendations for Treatment', in M. H. Ben-Aron, S. J. Hucker and C. D. Webster (eds), *Clinical Criminology*, M & M Graphics, Toronto, 1985

Abel, G. G., and Osborn, C., 'The Paraphilias: The Extent and Nature of Sexually Deviant and Criminal Behavior', in J. M. W. Bradford (ed.), *Psychiatric Clinics of North America*, 15:3, 675–87, September 1992

Abramson, P., and Pinkerton, S., *With Pleasure: Thoughts on the Nature of Human Sexuality*, OUP, Oxford, 1995

——, *Sexual Nature/Sexual Culture*, University of Chicago Press, Chicago, 1996

Ackerman, D., *A Natural History of Love*, Vintage, New York, 1994

Acton, W., *Prostitution, Considered in Its Moral, Social and Sanitary Aspects*, n.p., London, 1857

——, *The Functions and Disorders of the Reproductive Organs in Childhood, Youth, Adult Age, and Advanced Life, Considered in Their Physiological, Social, and Moral Relations*, Presley Blakiston, Philadelphia (PA), 1875

Adams, H. E., Davis, J. M., and Lohr, B. A., 'Sexual Arousal to Erotic and Aggressive Stimuli in Sexually Coercive and Noncoercive Men', *Journal of Abnormal Psychology*, 106:2, 230–42, 1997

Ainsworth, M. D. S., 'Attachment: Retrospect and Prospect', in C. M. Parkes and J. Stevenson-Hinde (eds), *The Place of Attachment in Human Behavior*, Basic Books, New York, 1982

——, 'Attachments Across the Life Span', *Bulletin of the New York Academy of Medicine*, 61, 792–811, 1985

Ainsworth, M. D. S., Blehar, M. C., Waters, E., and Wall, S., *Patterns of Attachment: A Psychological Study of the Strange Situation*, Erlbaum, Hillsdale (NJ), 1978

Alexander, R. D., *The Biology of Moral Systems*, Aldine de Gruyter, New York, 1987

Alexander, R. D., and Noonan, K. M., 'Concealment of Ovulation, Parental Care and Human Social Evolution', in N. Chagnon and W. Irons (eds), *Evolutionary Biology and Human Social Behavior*, Duxbury, North Scituate (MA), 1979

Allen, L. S., and Gorski, R. A., 'Sex Difference in the Bed Nucleus of the Stria Terminalis of the Human Brain', *Journal of Comparative Neurology*, 302:697–706, 1990

——, 'Sexual Dimorphism of the Anterior Commissure and Massa Intermedia of the Human Brain', *Journal of Comparative Neurology*, 312:97–104, 1991

——, 'Sexual Orientation and the Size of the Anterior Commissure in the Human Brain', *Proceedings of the National Academy of Sciences of the USA*, 89:7199–202, 1992

Allen, L. S., Richey, M. F., Chai, Y. M., and Gorski, R. A., 'Sex Differences in the Corpus Callosum of the Living Human Being', *Journal of Neuroscience*, 11:4, 933–42, 1991

Anonymous, *The Holy Bible* (King James Version), Harper, New York, 1995

——, *Onania; Or, the Heinous Sin of Self-Pollution, and All Its Frightful Consequences, in both Sexes, Considered. With Spiritual and Physical Advice to Those Who Have Already Injur'd Themselves by this Abominable Practice*, John Phillips, Boston (MA), 1724; facsimile reprint edition in C. Rosenberg and C. Smith-Rosenberg (eds), *The Secret Vice Exposed! Some Arguments Against Masturbation*, Arno Press, New York, 1974

Anthony, E., *Thy Rod and Staff: New Light on the Flagellatory Impulse*, Little Brown, London, 1995

Armstrong, K., *A History of God*, William Heinemann, London, 1993

Aron, A., 'The Matching Hypothesis Reconsidered: Comment on Kalick and Hamilton', *Journal of Personality and Social Psychology*, 54:3, 441–6, 1988

Aron, A., Aron, E. N., Tudor, M., and Nelson, G., 'Close Relationships as Including Others in the Self', *Journal of Personality and Social Psychology*, 60:2, 241–53, 1991

Aron, A., Aron, E. N., and Smollan, D., 'Inclusion of Other in the Self Scale and the Structure of Interpersonal Closeness', *Journal of Personality and Social Psychology*, 63:4, 596–612, 1992

Aron, A., Melinat, E., Aron, E. N., Vallone, R. D., and Bator, R. J., 'The Experimental Generation of Interpersonal Closeness: A Procedure and Some Preliminary Findings', *Personality and Social Psychology Bulletin*, 23:4, 363–77, 1997

Aron, A., and Westbay, L., 'Dimensions of the Prototype of Love', *Journal of Personality and Social Psychology*, 70:3, 535–51, 1996

Aron, E. N., and Aron, A., 'Love and Expansion of the Self: The State of the Model', *Personal Relationships*, 3:45–8, 1996

Augustine, St, *The Confessions of St Augustine*, Quality Paperback Club, New York, 1991

Bailey, J. M., Dunne, M., and Martin, N. G., 'Sex Differences in the Distribution and Determinants of Sexual Orientation', *Nature Genetics*, 1997 (under review)

Bailey, J. M., Finkel, E., Blackwelder, K., and Bailey, T., 'Masculinity, Femininity and Sexual Orientation', *Journal of Personality and Social Psychology*, 1997 (under review)

Bailey, J. M., Gaulin S., Agyei, Y., and Gladue, B. A., 'Effects of Gender and Sexual Orientation on Evolutionarily Relevant Aspects of Human Mating Psychology', *Journal of Personality and Social Psychology*, 66:6, 1081–93, 1994

Bailey, J. M., and Pillard, R., 'Genetics of Human Sexual Orientation', *The Annual Review of Sex Research*, 1996

Baker, R. R., *Sperm Wars: Infidelity, Sexual Conflict and Other Bedroom Battles*, Fourth Estate, London, 1996

Baker, R. R., and Bellis, M. A., '"Kamikaze" Sperm in Mammals?', *Animal Behaviour*, 33:1387–8, 1988

——, 'Elaboration of the Kamikaze Sperm Hypothesis: A Reply to Harcourt', *Animal Behaviour*, 37:865–7, 1989

——, 'Number of Sperm in Human Ejaculates Varies in Accordance with Sperm Competition', *Animal Behaviour*, 37:867–9, 1989

——, 'Human Sperm Competition: Ejaculate Manipulation by Females and a Function for Female Orgasm', *Animal Behaviour*, 46:887–909, 1993

——, *Human Sperm Competition: Copulation, Masturbation and Infidelity*, Chapman & Hall, New York, 1995

Bancroft, J., *Human Sexuality and Its Problems* (2nd edn), Churchill Livingstone, London, 1989

Barbaree, H. E., and Marshall, W. L., 'Erectile Responses Among Heterosexual Child Molesters, Father–Daughter Incest Offenders, and Matched Non-offenders: Five Distinct Age Preference Profiles', *Canadian Journal of Behavioral Science*, 21:1, 70–82, 1989

Barlow, D. H., Sakheim, D. K., and Beck, J. G., 'Anxiety Increases Sexual Arousal', *Journal of Abnormal Psychology*, 92, 49–54, 1983

Barkow, J. M., Cosmides, L., and Tooby, J. (eds), *The Adapted Mind*, OUP, New York, 1992

Barthes, R. (trs. R. Howard), *A Lover's Discourse: Fragments*, Penguin, London, 1990

Becker, J. B., Breedlove, S. M., and Crews, D., *Behavioral Endocrinology*, MIT Press, Cambridge (MA), 1993

Behrens, T., *The Monument*, Jonathan Cape, London, 1988

Bell, A. P., and Weinberg, S., *Homosexualities: A Study of Diversity Among Men and Women*, Simon & Schuster, New York, 1978

Bell, A. P, Weinberg, S., and Hammersmith, S. K., *Sexual Preference: Its Development in Men and Women*, Indiana University Press, Bloomington (IN), 1981

Bellis, M. A., and Baker, R. R., 'Do Females Promote Sperm Competition? Data for Humans', *Animal Behaviour*, 40:997–9, 1990

Benjamin, J., Lin, L., Patterson, C., et al, 'Population and Familial Association Between the D4 Dopamine Receptor Gene and Measures of Novelty Seeking', *Nature Genetics*, 12:81–4, 1996

Benshoof, L., and Thornhill, R., 'The Evolution of Monogamy and Concealed Ovulation in Humans', *Journal of Social and Biological Structures*, 2:95–106, 1979

Berenbaum, S. A., and Hines, M., 'Early Androgens are Related to Childhood Sex-typed Toy Preferences', *Psychological Science*, 3:203–6, 1992

Berlin, F. S., 'Sex Offenders: A Biomedical Perspective' in J. C. Greer and I.

R. Stuart (eds), *The Sexual Aggressor: Current Perspectives on Treatment*, Van Nostrand Reinhold Company, New York, 1983

Berman, M., Gladue, B., and Taylor, S., 'The Effects of Hormones, Type-A Behavior Pattern, and Provocation on Aggression in Men', *Motivation and Emotion*, 17:2, 125–38, 1993

Betzig, L. L., *Despotism and Differential Reproduction: A Darwinian View of History*, Aldine de Gruyter, New York, 1986

——, 'Causes of Conjugal Dissolution: A Cross-Cultural Study', *Current Anthropology*, 30:654, 676, 1989

——, 'Medieval Monogamy', *Journal of Family History*, Vol. 20, 2:181–216, 1990

——, 'History' in M. Maxwell (ed.), *The Sociobiological Imagination*, SUNY, Albany (NY), 1991

——, 'Roman Polygyny', *Ethology and Sociobiology*, 13:309–49, 1992

——, 'Roman Monogamy', *Ethology and Sociobiology*, 13:351–83, 1992

——, 'Sex, Succession and Stratification in the First Six Civilizations' in L. Ellis (ed.), *Social Stratification and Socioeconomic Equality*, Praeger, New York, 1993

——, 'Sex in History', *Michigan Today*, 26:1, March 1994

——, 'Wanting Women Isn't New; Getting Them Is, Very', *Politics and the Life Sciences*, 14:1, 24–37, 1995

Betzig, L. L., Borgerhoff Mulder, M., and Turke, P. (eds), *Human Reproductive Behaviour*, CUP, Cambridge, 1988

Betzig, L. L., and Turke, P., 'Those Who Can Do: Wealth, Status and Reproductive Success on Ifaluk', *Ethology and Sociobiology*, 6:79–87, 1985

Birkett, D., *Serpent in Paradise*, Picador, London, 1997

Blackwood, E. (ed.), *The Many Faces of Homosexuality: Anthropological Approaches to Homosexual Behavior*, Harrington Park Press, New York, 1986

Borgerhoff Mulder, M., 'The Relevance of the Polygyny Threshold Model to Humans', in C. G. N. Mascie-Taylor and A. J. Boyce (eds), *Human Mating Patterns*, CUP, Cambridge, 1988

——, 'Women's Strategies in Polygynous Marriage', *Human Nature*, 31:45–70, 1992

Bornemann, E., *Childhood Phases of Maturity*, Prometheus, Buffalo (NY), 1994

Bouhdiba, A., *Sexuality in Islam*, Routledge & Kegan Paul, London, 1985

Bowlby, J., *Attachment and Loss, Volume 1. Attachment*, Basic Books, New York, 1969

——, *Attachment and Loss, Volume 2. Separation: Anxiety and Anger*, Basic Books, New York, 1973

——, *The Making and Breaking of Affectional Bonds*, Tavistock, London 1979

——, *Attachment and Loss, Volume 3. Loss*, Basic Books, New York, 1980

Broude, G. J., and Greene, S. J., 'Cross-cultural Codes on Twenty Sexual Attitudes and Practices', *Ethnology*, 15:409–29, 1976

Brown, D., *Human Universals*, McGraw-Hill, New York, 1991

Brown, D., and Hotra, D., 'Are Prescriptively Monogamous Societies Effectively Monogamous?' in L. L. Betzig, M. Borgerhoff Mulder and P. Turke (eds), *Human Reproductive Behaviour*, CUP, Cambridge, 1988

Brown, P., *The Body and Society: Men, Women and Sexual Renunciation in Early Christianity*, Columbia University Press, New York, 1988

Brownmiller, S., *Against Our Will: Men, Women, and Rape*, Simon & Schuster, New York, 1975

Bullough, V. L., *Sexual Variance in Society and History*, University of Chicago Press, Chicago, 1976/Wiley Interscience Press, New York 1976

Bullough, V. L., and Bullough, B., *Sin, Sickness and Sanity: A History of Sexual Attitudes*, Garland Publishing, New York, 1977

——, *Human Sexuality: An Encyclopaedia*, Garland Publishing, New York 1994

——, *Science in the Bedroom: A History of Sex Research*, Basic Books, New York, 1994

——, *Sexual Attitudes: Myths and Realities*, Prometheus, Buffalo (NY) 1995

—— et al., *How I Got Into Sex*, Prometheus, Buffalo (NY), 1997

Bullough, V. L., Bullough, B., and Elias, J., *Gender Blending*, Prometheus Buffalo (NY), 1997

Bullough, V. L., and Brundage, J., *Sexual Practices and the Medieval Church* Prometheus, Buffalo (NY), 1982

Burr, C., *A Separate Creation: How Biology Makes Us Gay*, Bantam, London 1996

Burt, D. M., and Perrett, D. I., 'Perception of Age in Adult Caucasian Male Faces: Computer Graphic Manipulation of Shape and Information' *Proceedings of the Royal Society of London*, B, 259:137–43, 1995

——, 'Perceptual Asymmetries in Judgments of Facial Attractiveness, Age, Gender, Speech and Expression', *Neuropsychologia*, 35:5, 685–93, 1997

Buss, D., 'Love Acts: The Evolutionary Biology of Love', in R. Sternberg and M. Barnes (eds), *The Psychology of Love*, Yale University Press, New Haven, 1988

——, 'From Vigilance to Violence: Tactics of Mate Retention in American Undergraduates', *Ethology and Sociobiology*, 9, 291–317, 1988

——, 'Sex Differences in Human Mate Preferences: Evolutionary Hypotheses Tested in 37 Cultures', *Behavioural and Brain Sciences*, 12:1–49, 1989

——, 'Conflict Between the Sexes: Strategic Interference and the Evocation of Anger and Angst', *Journal of Personality and Social Psychology*, 56:5, 735–47, 1989

——, 'Mate Preference Mechanisms: Consequences for Partner Choice and Intrasexual Competition', in J. H. Barkow, L. Cosmides and J. Tooby (eds), *The Adapted Mind*, OUP, New York, 1992

——, *The Evolution of Desire: Strategies of Human Mating*, Basic Books, New York, 1994

—— *et al.*, 'Sex Differences in Jealousy: Evolution, Physiology and Psychology', *Psychological Science*, 3:251–255, 1992

Buss, D., and Dedden, L. A., 'Derogation of Competitors', *Journal of Social and Personal Relationships*, 7:395–422, 1990

Buss, D., and Greer, A., 'Tactics for Promoting Sexual Encounters', *Journal of Sex Research*, 31:3, 185–201, 1994

Buss, D., and Malamuth, N. M., *Sex, Power, Conflict: Evolutionary and Feminist Perspectives*, OUP, New York, 1996

Buss, D., and Schmitt, D. P., 'Sexual Strategies Theory: An Evolutionary Perspective on Human Mating', *Psychological Review*, 100:204–32, 1993

——, 'Strategic Self-Promotion and Competitor Derogation: Sex and Context Effects on the Perceived Effectiveness of Mate Attraction Tactics', *Journal of Personality and Social Psychology*, 70:6, 1996

Buunk, B. P, Angleitner, A., Oubaid, V., and Buss, D., 'Sex Differences in Jealousy in Evolutionary and Cultural Perspective: Tests from the Netherlands, Germany and the United States', *Psychological Science*, 1996

Buunk, B. P, Angleitner, A., Oubaid, V., Buss, D., and van Driel, B., *Variant Lifestyles and Relationships*, Sage Publications, London, 1989

Byrne, D., *The Attraction Paradigm*, Academic Press, New York, 1971

Byrne, D., and Kelley, K., *Alternative Approaches to the Study of Sexual Behaviour*, Erlbaum, Hillsdale (NJ), 1986

Byrne, D., and Murnen, S. K., 'Maintaining Loving Relationships' in R Sternberg and M. Barnes (eds), *The Psychology of Love*, Yale University Press, New Haven, 1988

Capellanus, A. (trs. J. Parry), *The Art of Courtly Love*, Columbia University Press, New York, 1986

Caplan, P., *The Cultural Construction of Sexuality*, Routledge & Kegan Paul London, 1987

Carrier, J. M., 'Homosexual Behaviour in Cross-cultural Perspective' in J Marmor (ed.), *Homosexual Behavior: A Modern Reappraisal*, Basic Books New York, 1980

Carter, C. S., 'Oxytocin and Sexual Behavior', *Neuroscience and Bio behavioral Reviews*, 16:131–44, 1992

——, 'Neuroendocrine Perspective on Social Attachment and Love' *Psychoneuroendocrinology*, 1997

—— et al., 'Adrenocorticoid Hormones and the Development and Expression of Mammalian Monogamy', *Annals of the New York Academy of Sciences* 771:82–9, 1995

——, 'Peptides, Steroids and Pair Bonding', *Annals of the New York Academy of Sciences*, 1997

Cashdan, E., 'Attracting Mates: Effects of Paternal Investment on Mate Attraction Strategies', *Ethology and Sociobiology*, 14, 1–24, 1993

——, 'Women's Mating Strategies', *Evolutionary Anthropology*, 5:4, 134–43 1996

Chagnon, N., 'Is Reproductive Success Equal in Egalitarian Societies?', in N. Chagnon and W. Irons (eds), *Evolutionary Biology and Human Social Behavior*, Duxbury, North Scituate (MA), 1979

Chagnon, N., Flinn, M. V., and Melancon, T. F., 'Sex-Ratio Variation Among the Yanomamö Indians', in N. Chagnon and W. Irons (eds) *Evolutionary Biology and Human Social Behavior*, Duxbury, North Scituate (MA), 1979

Chagnon, N., and Irons, W. (eds), *Evolutionary Biology and Human Social Behavior*, Duxbury, North Scituate (MA), 1979

Classen, C., Howes, D., and Synnott, A., *Aroma: The Cultural History o Smell*, Routledge & Kegan Paul, London, 1994

Cloninger, C. R., Adolfsson, R., and Svrakic, N., 'Mapping Genes fo Human Personality', *Nature Genetics*, 12:3–4, 1996

Concar, D., 'Sex and the Symmetrical Body', *New Scientist*, 22 April 1995

——, 'Sisters Are Doing It for Themselves', *New Scientist*, 17 August 1996

Cosmides, L., and Tooby, J., 'Cognitive Adaptations for Social Exchange', in J. H. Barkow, L. Cosmides and J. Tooby (eds), *The Adapted Mind*, OUP, New York, 1992

Craik, E. (ed), *Marriage and Property: Women and Marital Customs in History*, Aberdeen University Press, Aberdeen, 1991

Crenshaw, T., *The Alchemy of Love and Lust*, G. P. Puttnam's Sons, New York, 1996

Crenshaw, T., and Goldberg, J. P., *Sexual Pharmacology: Drugs That Affect Sexual Functioning*, W. W. Norton & Co., New York, 1996

Cronin, H., *The Ant and the Peacock*, CUP, Cambridge, 1993

Crow, T. J., 'Sexual Selection as the Mechanism of Evolution of Machiavellian Intelligence: A Darwinian Theory of the Origins of Psychosis', *Journal of Psychopharmacology*, 10:1, 77–87, 1996

Daly, M., Wilson, M., and Weghorst, S. J., 'Male Sexual Jealousy', *Ethology and Sociobiology*, 3:11–27, 1982

Daly, M., and Wilson, M., *Sex, Evolution and Behavior*, Willard Grant Press, Boston, 1983

——, *Homicide*, Aldine de Gruyter, New York, 1988

——, 'Killing the Competition: Female/Female and Male/Male Homicide', *Human Nature*, 1:81–107, 1990

——, 'The Man Who Mistook His Wife for a Chattel', in J. H. Barkow, L. Cosmides and J. Tooby (eds), *The Adapted Mind*, OUP, New York, 1992

Damasio, A., *Descartes' Error: Emotion, Reason and the Human Brain*, Grosset/Puttnam, New York, 1994

Darwin, C., *The Origin of Species by Means of Natural Selection, or the Preservation of Favoured Races in the Struggle for Life*, John Murray, London, 1859; reprinted by Mentor, New York

——, *The Descent of Man and Selection in Relation to Sex*, John Murray, London, 1871; Macmillan, London, 1883; reprinted by Princeton University Press, Princeton (MA), 1981

Dawkins, R., *The Selfish Gene*, OUP, Oxford, 1976

Dawkins, R., and Krebs, J. R., 'Arms Races Between and Within Species', *Proceedings of the Royal Society of London*, B, 205:489–511, 1979

de Beauvoir, S. (trs. and ed. H. M. Parshley), *The Second Sex*, Bantam, New York, 1961

D'Emilio, J., and Freedman, E., *Intimate Matters: A History of Sexuality in America*, Harper & Row, New York, 1988

de Rougemont, D., *Love in the Western World*, Pantheon, New York, 1956

Deacon, T., *The Symbolic Species: The Co-evolution of Language and the Human Brain*, Penguin Press, London, 1997

Diamond, J., *Why is Sex Fun? The Evolution of Human Sexuality*, Weidenfeld & Nicolson, London, 1997

Dickemann, M., 'The Ecology of Mating Systems in Hypergynous Dowry Societies', *Social Science Information*, 18:163–95, 1979

——, 'Female Infanticide and Reproductive Strategies of Stratified Human Societies' in N. Chagnon and W. Irons (eds), *Evolutionary Biology and Human Social Behavior*, Duxbury, North Scituate (MA), 1979

——, 'Paternal Confidence and Dowry Competition: A Biocultural Analysis of Purdah', in R. D. Alexander and D. W. Tinkle, *Natural Selection and Social Behavior: Recent Research and New Theory*, Chiron Press, New York, n.d.

——, 'Reproductive Strategies and Gender Construction: An Evolutionary View of Homosexualities', in J. P. de Cecco and J. P. Elia (eds), *If You Seduce a Straight Person, Can You Make Them Gay?*, Harrington Park Press, New York, 1993

——, 'Wilson's Panchreston: The Inclusive Fitness Hypothesis of Sociobiology Re-Examined', *Journal of Homosexuality*, 28:1/2, 147–83, Haworth Press, 1995

Dion, K. L., and Dion, K. K., 'Romantic Love: Individual and Cultural Perspectives', in R. Sternberg and M. Barnes (eds), *The Psychology of Love*, Yale University Press, New Haven, 1988

Dobash, R. P., and Dobash, R. E., 'Wives: The "Appropriate" Victims of Marital Violence', *Victimology*, 2:426–42, 1978

Dobash, R. P., Dobash, R. E., Cavanagh, C., and Wilson, M., 'Victimology Interview: Wife Beating – The Victims Speak', *Victimology*, 2:608–22, 1978

Dover K. J., *Greek Homosexuality*, Harvard University Press, Cambridge (MA), 1978

Duberman, M. B., Vicinus, M., and Chauncey, G. (eds), *Hidden from History: Reclaiming the Gay and Lesbian Past*, Penguin, London, 1989

Dunbar, R., 'Are You Lonesome Tonight?', *New Scientist*, 11 February 1995

Dutton, D., *The Batterer*, Basic Books, New York, 1995

——, 'Gender Differences in Anger/Anxiety Reactions to Witnessing Dyadic Family Conflict', *Canadian Journal of Behavioral Science*, 26:3, 353–64, 1994

Dutton, D., and Aron, A. P., 'Some Evidence for Heightened Sexual Attraction Under Conditions of High Anxiety', *Journal of Personality and Social Psychology*, 30:4, 510–17, 1974

Dutton, D., Saunders, K., and Starzomski, A., 'Intimacy-Anger and Insecure Attachment as Precursors of Abuse in Intimate Relationships', *Journal of Applied Social Psychology*, 24:15, 1367–86, 1994

Ebstein, R. P., Novick, O., Umansky, R., *et al.*, 'Dopamine D4 receptor (D4DR) Exon III Polymorphism Associated With the Human Personality Trait of Novelty Seeking', *Nature Genetics*, 12:78–80, 1996

Edelman, G. M., *Bright Air, Brilliant Fire: On the Matter of the Mind*, Allen Lane, London, 1992

Ellis, B., and Symons, D., 'Sex Differences in Sexual Fantasy: An Evolutionary Psychological Approach', *Journal of Sex Research*, 25: 527–55, 1990

Ellis, H., *Studies in the Psychology of Sex*, F. A. Davies, New York, 1905; reprinted by Random House, New York, 1942

Everaerd, W., and Laan E., 'Desire for Passion: Energetics of Sexual Response', *Journal of Sex and Marital Therapy*, 21:4, 355–63, 1995

Faderman, L., *Surpassing the Love of Men* (3rd edn), The Women's Press, London, 1985

Farrar, F. W., *The Life of St Augustine*, Hodder & Stoughton, London, 1993

Fisher, H. E., 'The Four-year Itch', *Natural History*, 22–23 October 1987

——, 'Evolution of Human Serial Pairbonding', *American Journal of Physical Anthropology*, 78:331–54, 1989

——, 'Monogamy, Adultery and Divorce in Cross-species Perspective', in M. H. Robinson and L. Tiger (eds), *Man and Beast Revisited*, Smithsonian Institution Press, Washington DC, 1991

——, *Anatomy of Love: The Natural History of Monogamy, Adultery and Divorce*, W. W. Norton & Co., New York, 1992

——, 'The Nature of Romantic Love', *The Journal of NIH Research*, 6: 59–64, 1994

——, 'The Nature and Evolution of Romantic Love', in W. Jankowiak (ed.), *Romantic Passion: A Universal Experience?*, Columbia University Press, New York, 1995

Ford, C. S., and Beach, F. A., *Patterns of Sexual Behaviour*, Harper & Row, New York, 1951

Foster, L., *Religion and Sexuality: Three American Communal Experiments of the Nineteenth Century*, OUP, Oxford, 1981

Forsyth, A., *A Natural History of Sex*, Chapters Publishing, Shelburne (VT), 1996

Foucault, M. (trs. R. Hurley), *The History of Sexuality. Volumes 1–3*, Vintage, New York, 1985

Fox, R., *The Red Lamp of Incest*, Dutton, New York, 1980

Frayser, S. G., *Varieties of Sexual Experience: An Anthropological Perspective on Human Sexuality*, HRAF Press, New Haven, 1985

——, *Studies in Human Sexuality: A Selected Guide*, HRAF Press, New Haven, 1987

Friday, N., *My Secret Garden: Women's Sexual Fantasies*, Quartet, London, 1973

——, *Forbidden Flowers*, Pocket Books, New York, 1975

——, *Men in Love*, Bantam, New York, 1980

Gallup Jr, G. G., and Suarez, D., 'Homosexuality as a By-product of Selection for Optimal Heterosexual Strategies', *Perspectives in Biology and Medicine*, 26:315–22, 1983

Gamman, L., and Makinen, M., *Female Fetishism: A New Look*, Lawrence & Wishart, London, 1994

Garber, M., *Vice Versa: Bisexuality and the Eroticism of Everyday Life*, Hamish Hamilton, London, 1996

Gaylin, W., and Person, E., *Passionate Attachments*, The Free Press, New York, 1988

Geer, J. H., and O'Donohue, W. (eds), *Theories of Human Sexuality*, Plenum Press, New York, 1987

Gerlsma, C., Buunk, B. P., and Musters, W. C., 'Correlates of Self-reported Adult Attachment Styles in a Dutch Sample of Married Men and Women', *Journal of Social and Personal Relationships*, 13:2, 313–20 1996

Gibson, I., *The English Vice: Beating, Sex and Shame in Victorian England and After*, Duckworth, London, 1979

Gilbert, H., *The Sexual Imagination: From Acker to Zola*, Jonathan Cape London, 1993

Gillis, J. R., 'From Ritual to Romance: Toward an Alternative History c

Love', in C. Stearns and P. Stearns (eds), *Emotion and Social Change*, n.p., New York, 1988

Gladue, B. A., 'The Biopsychology of Sexual Orientation', *Current Directions in Psychological Science*, 3:5,150–4, 1994

Gladue, B. A., Beatty, W. W., Larson, J., and Staton, R. D., 'Sexual Orientation and Spatial Ability in Men and Women', *Psychobiology*, 18:1, 101–8, 1990

Gladue, B. A., Boechler, M., and McCaul, K. D., 'Hormonal Response to Competition in Human Males', *Aggressive Behavior*, 15, 409–22, 1989

Gladue, B. A., and Delany, J. J., 'Gender Differences in Perception of Attractiveness of Men and Women in Bars', *Personality and Social Psychology Bulletin*, 16, 378–91, 1990

Gooren, L. J., 'Concepts and Methods of Biomedical Research into Homosexuality and Transsexualism', *Journal of Psychology and Human Sexuality*, 6:1, 5–21, 1993

Gooren, L. J., and Cohen-Kettenis, P. T., 'Development of Male Gender/Identity Role and a Sexual Orientation Towards Women in a 46 XY Subject with an Incomplete Form of the Androgen Insensitivity Syndrome', *Archives of Sexual Behavior*, 20:5, 459–70, 1991

Gooren, L. J., Fliers, E., and Courtney, K., 'Biological Determinants of Sexual Orientation', *Annual Review of Sex Research*, 1:175–96, 1990

Gottman, J. M., 'Predicting the Longitudinal Course of Marriages', *Journal of Marital and Family Therapy*, 17:1, 1991

——, *What Predicts Divorce*, Erlbaum, Hillsdale (NJ), 1994

——, *Why Marriages Succeed or Fail*, Simon & Schuster, New York, 1994

Graham, S., *A Lecture to Young Men*, Weedon & Cory, Providence, 1834; facsimile reprint edition by Arno Press, New York, 1974

Grammer, K., Filova, V., and Fieder, M., 'The communication Paradox and Possible Solutions: Towards a Radical Empiricism' (no date or publication details)

Grammer, K., Jütte, A., and Fischermann, B., 'The Fight Between the Sexes . . . and the War of the Signals', in *Sexualität im Spiegel der Wissenschaft: Edition Universitas*, Hirzel, Stuttgart, 1996

Green, R., 'Gender Identity in Childhood and Later Sexual Orientation', *American Journal of Psychiatry*, 142: 339–41, 1985

——, *The 'Sissy-Boy Syndrome' and the Development of Homosexuality*, Yale University Press, New Haven, 1987

Greenberg, D. F., *The Construction of Homosexuality*, University of Chicago Press, Chicago, 1988

Greenberg, M., and Littlewood, R., 'Post-adoption Incest and Phenotypic Matching: Experience, Personal Meanings and Biosocial Implications', *British Journal of Medical Psychology*, 68:29–44, 1995

Gregersen, E., *The World of Human Sexuality*, Irvington, New York, 1994

Gutierres, S. E., Kenrick, D. T., and Partch, J. J., 'Contrast Effects in Self-assessment Reflect Evolved Gender Differences in Mating Criteria', 1997 (in press)

Hamer, D. H., and Copeland, P., *Science of Desire: The Search for the Gay Gene and the Biology of Behaviour*, Simon & Schuster, New York, 1994

Hamer, D. H., Hu, S., Magnuson, V., *et al.*, 'A Linkage Between DNA Markers on the X Chromosome and Male Sexual Orientation', *Science*, 261:321–7, 1993

Hamilton, W. D., 'The Evolution of Altruistic Behaviour', *American Naturalist*, 97:354–6, 1963

——, 'The Genetical Evolution of Social Behaviour', Parts 1 and 2, *Journal of Theoretical Biology*, 7:1–52, 1964

——, 'Extraordinary Sex Ratios', *Science*, 156:477–88, 1967

——, 'Gamblers Since Life Began: Barnacles, Aphids, Elms', review of Williams' *Evolution of Sex* and Ghiselin's *The Economy of Nature and the Evolution of Sex*, in *Quarterly Review of Biology*, 50:175–80, 1975

——, 'Sex Versus Non-Sex Versus Parasite', *Oikos*, 35:282–90, 1980

——, 'Recurrent Viruses and Theories of Sex', *TREE*, 7:8, 277–8, 1992

Hamilton, W. D., Axelrod, R., and Tanese, R., 'Sexual Reproduction as an Adaptation to Resist Parasites', *Proceedings of the National Academy of Sciences of the USA*, 87:3566–73, 1990

Harper, R.F., *The Code of Hammurabi, King of Babylon About 2250 BC* University of Chicago Press, Chicago, 1904

Harris, H., *Human Nature and the Nature of Romantic Love*, 1995 (manuscript)

Harrison, B., 'Underneath the Victorians', *Victorian Studies*, 10:3, 239–63 1966–67

Harrison, F., *The Dark Angel: Aspects of Victorian Sexuality*, Fontana London, 1977

Haste, C., *Rules of Desire: Sex in Britain, World War I to the Present*, Pimlico London, 1992

Hatfield, E., 'Passionate Love and Companionate Love', in R. Sternberg and M. Barnes (eds), *The Psychology of Love*, Yale University Press, New Haven, 1988

Hatfield, E., and Clark, R. D., 'Gender Differences in Receptivity to Sexual Offers', *Journal of Psychology and Human Sexuality*, 2:1, 39–55, 1989

Hatfield, E., and Rapson, R. L., *Love, Sex and Intimacy: Their Psychology, Biology and History*, HarperCollins, New York, 1993

Hatfield, E., Sprecher, S., Pillemer, J. T., Greenberger, D., and Wexler, P., 'Gender Differences in What Is Desired in the Sexual Relationship', *Journal of Psychology and Human Sexuality*, 1:2, 39–52, 1988

Hauspfater, G., and Hrdy, S. B., *Infanticide: Comparative and Evolutionary Perspectives*, Aldine Press, New York, 1984

Hazan, C., and Shaver, P., 'Attachment as an Organizational Framework for Research on Human Relationships', *Psychological Inquiry*, 5:1, 1–22, 1994

———, 'Deeper Into Attachment Theory', *Psychological Inquiry*, 5:1, 68–79, 1994

Heiman, J. R., 'Female Sexual Response Patterns', *Archives of General Psychiatry*, 37: 1311–16, 1980

———, 'A Process Model of Adult Attachment Formation', in *Handbook of Personal Relationships* (2nd edn), John Wiley, New York, 1997

Heiman, J. R., and Morokoff, P. J., 'Effects of Erotic Stimuli on Sexually Functional and Dysfunctional Women: Multiple Measures Before and After Sex Therapy', *Behavioural Research and Therapy*, 18:127–37, 1980

Heiman, J. R., and Rowland, D. L., 'Affective and Physiological Sexual Response Patterns: The Effects of Instructions on Sexually Functional and Dysfunctional Men', *Journal of Psychosomatic Research*, 27:2, 105–16, 1983

Heiman, J. R., Rowland, D. L., Hatch, J. P., and Gladue, B. A., 'Psychophysiological and Endocrine Responses to Sexual Arousal in Women', *Archives of Sexual Behavior*, 20:2, 171–86, 1991

Henriques, F., *Love in Action: The Sociology of Sex*, Dutton, New York, 1960

———, *The Pretence of Love: Prostitution and Society. Volume I: Primitive, Classical and Oriental*, Panther, London, 1962

Hill, E. M., Nocks, E. S., and Gardner, L., 'Physical Attractiveness: Manipulation by Physique and Status Displays', *Ethology and Sociobiology*, 8:143–54, 1987

Hines, M., Chiu, L., McAdams, L. A., Bentler, P. M., and Lipcamon, J., 'Cognition and the Corpus Callosum: Verbal Fluency, Visuospatial Ability and Language Lateralization Related to Midsagittal Surface Areas of Callosal Subregions', *Behavioral Neuroscience*, 106: 3–14, 1992

Hinsch, B., *Passions of the Cut Sleeve: The Male Homosexual Tradition in China*, University of California Press, London, 1990

Hite, S., *The Hite Report on Female Sexuality*, Dell, New York, 1976

——, *The Hite Report on Male Sexuality*, Ballantine, New York, 1981

Hofman, M. A., and Swaab, D. F., 'The Sexually Dimorphic Nucleus of the Preoptic Area in the Human Brain: A Comparative Morphometric Study', *Journal of Anatomy*, 164: 55–72, 1989

Hrdy, S. B., 'Infanticide Among Animals: A Review, Classification and Examination of the Implications for the Reproductive Strategies of Females', *Ethology and Sociobiology*, 1:13–40, 1979

——, 'The Evolution of Human Sexuality: The Latest Word and the Last', review of Symons' *Evolution of Human Sexuality*, in *The Quarterly Review of Biology*, 54:309–14, 1979

——, *The Woman That Never Evolved*, Harvard University Press, Cambridge, 1981

——, 'Behavioral Biology and the Double Standard', in S. K. Wasser (ed.), *Social Behavior of Female Vertebrates*, Academic Press, New York, 1983

——, 'Empathy, Polyandry, and the Myth of the Coy Female', in R. Bleier (ed.), *Feminist Approaches to Science*, Pergamon Press, New York, 1986

——, 'The Primate Origins of Human Sexuality', in R. Bellig and G. Stevens (eds), *The Evolution of Sex*, record of Nobel Conference XXIII, Harper & Row, San Francisco, 1988

——, 'Sex Bias in Nature and in History: A Late 1980s Re-examination of the "Biological Origins" Argument', *Yearbook of Physical Anthropology*, 33:25–37, 1990

Hrdy, S. B., Janson, C., and Schaik, C., 'Infanticide: Let's Not Throw Out the Baby With the Bath Water', *Evolutionary Anthropology*, 8:5 1994–95

Hrdy, S. B., and Whitten, P. L., 'Patterning of Sexual Activity', in B. Smuts *et al.* (eds), *Primate Societies*, University of Chicago Press, Chicago 1987

Hu, S., Pattatucci, M., Patterson, C., *et al.*, 'Linkage Between Sexual Orientation and Chromosome Xq28 in Males but not in Females *Nature Genetics*, 11:248–56, 1995

Hucker, S. J., 'Self-harmful Sexual Behavior', *Psychiatric Clinics of North America*, 8:2, 323–37, 1985

Hucker, S. J., Langevin, R., Wortzman, G., Bain, J., Handy, L., Chambers, J., and Wright, S., 'Neuropsychological Impairment in Pedophiles', *Canadian Journal of Behavioral Science*, 18, 440–8, 1986

Hucker, S. J. and Stermac, L., 'The Evaluation and Treatment of Sexual Violence, Necrophilia and Asphyxiophilia', *Psychiatric Clinics of North America*, 15:3, 703–19, 1992

Hull, E. M., Lorrain, D. S., and Matuszewich, L., 'Extracellular Dopamine in the Medial Preoptic Area: Implications of Sexual Motivation and Hormonal Control of Copulation', *The Journal of Neuroscience*, 15:11, 7465–71, 1995

—— *et al.*, 'Organisational and Activational Effects of Dopamine on Male Sexual Behavior', in L. Ellis and L. Ebertz (eds), *Males, Females and Behavior: Toward Biological Understanding*, Praeger Press, Westport (CT), 1998

Hunt, M. J., *The Natural History of Love*, Hutchinson, London, 1960

Insel, T. R., and Carter, C. S., 'The Monogamous Brain . . .', *Natural History*, August 1995

Irons, R., 'Human Female Reproductive Strategies' in S. K. Wasser (ed), *Social Behavior of Female Vertebrates*, Academic Press, New York, 1985

Jackson, J. C., *Hints on the Reproductive Organs: Their Diseases, Causes and Cure on Hydropathic Principles*, Fowlers & Wells, Boston (MA), 1853

——, *The Sexual Organism and Its Healthful Management*, B. Leverett Emerson, Boston (MA), 1865

Jankowiak, W., *Sex, Death and Hierarchy in a Chinese City: An Anthropological Account*, Columbia University Press, New York, 1992

——, *Romantic Passion: A Universal Experience*, Columbia University Press, New York, 1994

Jankowiak, W., and Fischer, E. F., 'A Cross-cultural Perspective on Romantic Love', *Ethnology*, 31:2: 149–55, 1992

Johnson, R. A., *We: Understanding the Psychology of Romantic Love*, Harper & Row, San Francisco, 1983

Johnston, V. S., and Franklin, M., 'Is Beauty in the Eye of the Beholder?', *Ethology and Sociobiology*, 14: 183–99, 1993

Jordan, H. W., and Howe, G., 'De Clérambault Syndrome (Erotomania):

A Review and Case Presentation', *Journal of the National Medical Association*, 72:10, 979–85, 1980

Jordan, H. W., and Johnson-Warren, M., 'Erotomania: Seventeen Years Later', 1997

Kalish, N., *Lost and Found Lovers*, Morrow, New York, 1997

Kaplan, L. J., *Female Perversions*, Penguin, London, 1991

Karlen, A., 'Homosexuality in History', in J. Marmor (ed.), *Homosexual Behavior: A Modern Reappraisal*, Basic Books, New York, 1980

Katz, J. N., *The Invention of Heterosexuality*, Plume Books, New York, 1995

Kellogg, J. H., *Man the Masterpiece, or Plain Truths Plainly Told about Boyhood, Youth, and Manhood*, Signs of the Times Publishing Association, Warburton (Australia), 1906

——, *Plain Facts for Old and Young, Embracing the Natural History and Hygiene of Organic Life*, I. F. Segner, Burlington (IA), 1888; facsimile reprint edition by Arno Press, New York, 1974

——, *The Ladies' Guide in Health and Disease: Girlhood, Maidenhood, Wifehood, Motherhood*, Signs of the Times Publishing Association, Warburton (Australia), 1908

Kennedy, J. G., 'Circumcision and Excision in Egyptian Nubia', *Man*, NS 5.2:175–91, 1970

Kenrick, D. T., and Gutierres, S. E., 'Contrast Effects and Judgments of Physical Attractiveness: When Beauty Becomes a Social Problem', *Journal of Personality and Social Psychology*, 38:1, 131–40, 1980

——, 'Influence of Popular Erotica on Judgements of Strangers and Mates', *Journal of Experimental Social Psychology*, 25, 159–67, 1989

——, 'Contrast Effects in Self-Assessment Reflect Evolved Gender Differences in Mating Criteria' (in press)

Kenrick, D. T., and Keefe, R. C., 'Age Preferences in Mates Reflect Sex Differences in Human Reproductive Strategies', *Behavioral and Brain Sciences*, 15, 75–133, 1992

Kenrick, D. T., Keefe, R. C., *et al.*, 'Age Preferences and Mate Choice Among Homosexuals and Heterosexuals: A Case for Modular Psychological Mechanisms', *Journal of Personality and Social Psychology*, 69:6, 1166–72, 1995

——, 'Adolescents' Age Preferences for Dating Partners: Support for an Evolutionary Model of Life-History Strategies', *Child Development*, 67, 1499–511, 1996

Kenrick, D. T., Neuberg, S. L, Zierk, K. L., and Krones, J. M., 'Evolution and Social Cognition: Contrast Effects as a Function of Sex, Dominance and Physical Attractiveness', *Personality and Social Psychology Bulletin*, 20:2, April 1994

Kenrick, D. T., Groth, G. E., Trost, M. R., and Sadalla, E. K., 'Integrating Evolutionary and Social Exchange Perspectives on Relationships: Effects of Gender, Self-appraisal and Involvement Level on Mate Selection Criteria', *Journal of Personality and Social Psychology*, 64:6, 951–69, 1993

Keuls, E. C., *The Reign of the Phallus: Sexual Politics in Ancient Athens*, University of California Press, London, 1985

King, B. M., *Human Sexuality Today*, Prentice Hall, New Jersey, 1996

Kinsey, A. C., Pomeroy, W. B., and Martin, C. E., *Sexual Behaviour in the Human Male*, W. B. Saunders, Philadelphia, 1948

Kinsey, A. C., Pomeroy, W. B., Martin, C. E., and Gebhard, P. H., *Sexual Behaviour in the Human Female*, W. B. Saunders, Philadelphia, 1953

Klassen, A. D., Williams, C. J., and Levitt, E. E, *Sex and Morality in the United States: An Empirical Enquiry Under the Auspices of the Kinsey Institute*, Wesleyan University Press, Middletown (CT), 1989

Klima, B., 'A Triple Burial from the Upper Palaeolithic of Dolni Vestonice, Czechoslovakia', *Journal of Human Evolution*, 16:831–5, 1988

Kohl, J. V., and Francoeur, R. T., *The Scent of Eros: Mysteries of Odor in Human Sexuality*, Continuum, New York, 1995

Kosnick, A., *et al.* (eds), *Human Sexuality: New Directions in American Catholic Thought*, Paulist Press, New York, 1977

Krafft-Ebing, R. von, *Psychopathia Sexualis* (translated from the 7th enlarged edition by C. G. Chaddock), F. A. Davis, Philadelphia, 1894

Kressel, G. M., 'Sororicide/Filiacide: Homicide for Family Honour', *Current Anthropology*, 22:2, 141–58, 1981

Kurosawa, M., Lundeberg, T., Agren, G., Lend, I., and Uvnas-Moberg, K., 'Massage-like Stroking of the Abdomen Lowers Blood Pressure in Anesthetized Rats: Influence of Oxytocin', *Journal of the Autonomic Nervous System*, 56, 26–30, 1995

Laan, E., and Everaerd, W., 'Determinants of Female Sexual Arousal: Psychophysiological Theory and Data', *Annual Review of Sex Research*, 6, 32–76, 1995

——, 'Habituation of Female Sexual Arousal to Slides and Film', *Archives of Sexual Behavior*, 24:5, 517–41, 1995

Laan, E., Everaerd, W., and Evers, A., 'Assessment of Female Sexua
Arousal: Response Specificity and Construct Validity', *Psychophysiology*
32, 476–85, 1995

Laan, E., Everaerd, W., van Aanhold, M., and Rebel, M., 'Performanc
Demand and Sexual Arousal in Women', *Behavioural Research an
Therapy*, 31:1, 25–35, 1993

Laan, E., Everaerd, W., van Bellen, G., and Hanewald, G., 'Women's Sex
ual and Emotional Responses to Male- and Female-Produced Erotica
Archives of Sexual Behavior, 23:2, 153–69, 1994

Laan, E., Everaerd, W., van Berlo, R., and Rijs, L., 'Mood and Sexua
Arousal in Women', *Behavioral Research and Therapy*, 33:4, 441–3
1995

La Cerra, P., Cosmides, L., and Tooby, J., 'Psychological Adaptations i
Women for Assessing a Man's Willingness to Invest in Offspring', pape
presented at the Fifth Annual Meeting of the Human Behavior an
Evolution Society, Binghamton, New York, 1993

Laiou, A. E. (ed.), *Consent and Coercion to Sex and Marriage in Ancient an
Medieval Societies*, Dumbarton Oaks, Washington DC, 1993

Langevin, R., 'Sexual Anomalies and the Brain', in W. L. Marshall, D
R. Laws and H. E. Barbaree (eds), *Handbook of Sexual Assault: Issue
Theories, and Treatment of the Offender*, Plenum Press, New York, 199(

Langfeldt, T., 'Sexual Development in Children', in M. Cook and K
Howells (eds), *Adult Sexual Interest in Children*, Academic Press, Londor
1981

Langlois, J. H., Ritter, J. M., Roggman, L. A., and Vaughn, L. S., 'Facia
Diversity and Infant Preferences for Attractive Faces', *Developmentc
Psychology*, 27:1, 79–84, 1991

Langlois, J. H., and Roggman, L. A., 'Attractive Faces Are Only Average
Psychological Science, 1, 115–21, 1990

Langlois, J. H., and Musselman, L., 'What is Average and What is Nc
Average About Attractive Faces?', *Psychological Science*, 5:4, 214–19
1994

——, 'The Myths and Mysteries of Beauty', in D. R. Calhoun (ed.]
1996 Yearbook of Science and the Future, Encyclopaedia Britannica
Chicago, 1996

Langlois, J. H., and Rieser-Danner, L. A., 'Infants' Differential Socia
Responses to Attractive and Unattractive Faces', *Developmental Psychol
ogy*, 26:1, 153–9, 1990

Lake, M., *Scents and Sensuality: The Essence of Excitement*, John Murray, London, 1989

Laqueur, T., *Making Sex: Body and Gender from the Greeks to Freud*, Harvard University Press, Cambridge (MA), 1992

Laumann, E. O., Gagnon, J. H., *et al.*, *The Social Organization of Sexuality: Sexual Practices in the United States*, University of Chicago Press, Chicago, 1994

Lawson, A., *Adultery: An Analysis of Love and Betrayal*, Basic Books, New York, 1988

Legg, C. R., and Booth, D. (eds), *Appetite: Neural and Behavioural Bases*, OUP, Oxford, 1994

Leitenberg, H., and Henning, K., 'Sexual Fantasy', *Psychological Bulletin*, 117:3, 469–96, 1995

Lesch, K. P., Bengel, D., Heils, A., *et al.*, 'Association of Anxiety-related Traits with a Polymorphism in the Serotonin Transporter Gene Regulatory Region', *Science*, 274:1527–30, 29 November 1996

Levin, R. J., 'Facets of Female Behaviour Supporting the Social Script Model of Human Sexuality', *Journal of Sex Research*, 11:4, 348–52, 1975

——, 'The Mechanics of Human Female Sexual Arousal', *Annual Review of Sex Research*, 3, 1–47, 1992

Levin, R. J., and Wagner, G., 'Self-reported Central Sexual Arousal Without Vaginal Arousal, Duplicity or Veracity Revealed by Objective Measurement', *Journal of Sex Research*, 540–4, n.d.

Lewinsohn, R., *A History of Sexual Customs*, Harper, New York, 1958

Lewis, C. S., *The Allegory of Love*, OUP, Oxford, 1938

LeVay, S., *The Sexual Brain*, MIT Press, Cambridge (MA), 1993

Liebowitz, M. R., *The Chemistry of Love*, Little, Brown, Boston (MA), 1983

Littlewood, R., 'Military Rape', *Anthropology Today*, 13:2, 7–16, 1997

Lytle Croutier, A., *Harem: The World Behind the Veil*, Bloomsbury, London, 1989

Macfarlane, A., *Marriage and Love in England, 1300–1840*, Blackwell, Oxford, 1986

MacLean, P. D., *A Triune Concept of the Brain and Behaviour*, University of Toronto Press, Toronto, 1973

——, 'Sensory and Perceptive Factors in Emotional Function of the Triune

Brain' in R. G. Grennell and S. Gabay (eds), *Biological Foundations of Psychiatry*, Vol. 1, 177–98, 1976

——, 'Evolutionary Psychiatry and the Triune Brain', *Psychological Medicine*, 15, 219–21, 1985

McWhirter, D. P., Sanders, S. A., and Reinisch, J. M. (eds), *Homosexuality/Heterosexuality: Concepts of Sexual Orientation*, OUP, New York, 1990

Malamuth, N. M., 'Rape Proclivity Among Males', *Journal of Social Issues*, 37, 138–57, 1981

——, 'Evolution and Laboratory Research on Men's Sexual Arousal: What Do the Data Show and How Can We Explain Them', *Behavioral and Brain Sciences*, 15, 394–6, 1992

——, 'The Confluence Model of Sexual Aggression: Feminist and Evolutionary Perspectives', in D. Buss and N. M. Malamuth (eds), *Sex, Power, Conflict: Evolutionary and Feminist Perspectives*, OUP, New York, 1996

Malinowski, B., *The Sexual Life of Savages in North-Western Melanesia*, Routledge & Sons, London, 1932

——, *Sex and Repression in Savage Society*, World, New York, 1965

Mandelker, I. L., *Religion, Society and Utopia in Nineteenth-Century America*, University of Massachusetts Press, Amherst, 1984

Manning, J. T., *et al.*, 'Asymmetry and the Menstrual Cycle in Women', *Ethology and Sociobiology*, 17:1–15, 1996

Marmor, J. (ed.), *Homosexual Behavior: A Modern Reappraisal*, Basic Books, New York, 1980

Marshall, D. S., and Suggs, R. C. (eds), *Human Sexual Behavior: Variations in the Ethnographic Spectrum*, Prentice Hall, New Jersey, 1972

Marshall, W. L., Laws, D. R., and Barbaree, H. E. (eds), *Handbook of Sexual Assault: Issues, Theories and Treatment of the Offender*, Plenum Press, New York, 1990

Mason, M., *The Making of Victorian Sexual Attitudes*, OUP, Oxford, 1994

Masters, W. H., and Johnson, V. E., *Human Sexual Response*, Little, Brown, Boston (MA), 1966

——, *Human Sexual Inadequacy*, Little, Brown, Boston (MA), 1970

——, *Homosexuality in Perspective*, Little, Brown, Boston (MA), 1979

Masters, W. H., Johnson, V. E., and Kolodny, R. C., *Masters and Johnson on Sex and Human Loving*, Little, Brown, Boston (MA), 1985

Matthews, M., *The Horseman: Obsessions of a Zoophile*, Prometheus, Buffalo (NY), 1994

Maynard Smith, J., 'What Use is Sex?', *Journal of Theoretical Biology*, 30:319–35, 1971

——, 'Recombination and the Rate of Evolution', *Genetics*, 78:299–304, 1974

——, 'Why Be an Hermaphrodite?', *Nature*, 263:125–6, 1976

——, *The Evolution of Sex*, CUP, Cambridge, 1978

——, 'Contemplating Life Without Sex', *Nature*, 324:300–1, 1986

——, 'Theories of Sexual Selection', *Trends in Ecology and Evolution*, 6:146–1991

——, *The Major Transitions in Evolution*, W. H. Freeman, Oxford, 1995

McCaul, K. D., Gladue, B. A., and Joppa, M., 'Winning, Losing, Mood and Testosterone', *Hormones and Behavior*, 26, 486–504, 1992

McManners, J. (ed.), *The Oxford History of Christianity*, OUP, Oxford, 1993

Mead, M., *Coming of Age in Samoa*, Penguin, London, 1954

Mellen, S. L. W., *The Evolution of Love*, W. H. Freeman, San Francisco, 1981

Meston, C. M., and Gorzalka, B. B., 'Psychoactive Drugs and Human Sexual Behavior: The Role of Serotogenic Activity', *Journal of Psychoactive Drugs*, 24:1, 1–40, 1992

——, 'The Effects of Sympathetic Activation on Physiological and Subjective Sexual Arousal in Women', *Behavioral Research and Therapy*, 33:6, 651–64, 1995

Michod, R. E., and Levin, R. B. (eds), *The Evolution of Sex: An Examination of Current Ideas*, Sinauer Press, Sunderland (MA), 1987

Miller, G. F., 'Sexual Selection for Protean Expressiveness: A New Model of Hominid Encephalization', paper delivered to the 4th annual meeting of the Human Behaviour and Evolution Society, Alberquerque, 6–22 July 1992

Min, Anchee, *Red Azalea*, Victor Gollancz, London, 1993

Mithen, S., *The Prehistory of the Mind*, Thames & Hudson, London, 1996

Moir, A., and Jessel, D., *Brainsex: The Real Difference Between Men and Women*, Mandarin, London, 1989

Mondimore, F. M., *A Natural History of Homosexuality*, Johns Hopkins University Press, Baltimore, 1996

Money, J., *Love and Love Sickness*, Johns Hopkins University Press, Baltimore, 1980

——, *The Destroying Angel*, Prometheus, Buffalo (NY), 1985

——, *Gay, Straight and In-Between: The Sexology of Erotic Orientation*, OUP, Oxford, 1988

——, *Lovemaps*, Irvington, New York, 1988–93

——, *Reinterpreting the Unspeakable: Human Sexuality 2000*, Continuum, New York, 1994

——, *Gendermaps: Social Constructionism, Feminism and Sexosophical History*, Continuum, New York, 1995

——, *Principles of Developmental Sexology*, Continuum, New York, 1997

Money, J., Cawte, J. E., Bianchi, G. N., and Nurcombe, B., 'Sex Training and Traditions in Arnhem Land', *British Journal of Medical Psychology*, 43:383–99, 1970

Money, J., and Ehrhardt, A. A., *Man and Woman, Boy and Girl: The Differentiation and Dimorphism of Gender Identity from Conception to Maturity*, Johns Hopkins University Press, Baltimore, 1972

Money, J., and Lamacz, M., *Vandalized Lovemaps*, Prometheus, Buffalo (NY), 1989

Money, J., Wainwright, G., and Hingsburger, D., *The Breathless Orgasm: A Lovemap Biography of Asphyxiophilia*, Prometheus, Buffalo (NY), 1991

Muller-Lyer, F. C., *The Evolution of Modern Marriage*, Allen & Unwin, London 1913

Muncey, R. L., *Sex and Marriage in Utopian Communities: Nineteenth-century America*, Indiana University Press, Bloomington, 1973

Murphy, W. D., Seckl, J. R., Burton, S., Checkley, S. A., and Lightman, S. L., 'Changes in Oxytocin and Vasopressin Secretion During Sexual Activity in Men', *Journal of Clinical Endocrinology and Metabolism*, 65: 738–41, 1987

Murray, T. B., *Pitcairn: The Island, the People and the Pastor*, SPCK, London, 1853

——, *The Home of the Mutineers*, American Sunday School Union, Philadelphia, 1856

Nash, E., *Plaisirs d'Amour: An Erotic Guide to the Senses*, Harper San Francisco, New York, 1995

Nash, R. J., *Look for the Woman*, Harrap, London, 1984

Nefzawi, Sheikh (trs. R. Burton), *The Perfumed Garden*, Park Street Press, Rochester (VT), 1992

Neumann, F., 'Ulrich von Lichtenstein's Frauendienst', in *Zeitschrift für Deutschkunde*, 1926

Nicholson, R. B., *The Pitcairners*, Angus & Robertson, London, 1966

Ovid, *The Art of Love: Ovid's Ars Amatoria With Verse Translation by B. P. Moore*, n.p., London, 1935

Pagels, E., *Adam, Eve and the Serpent*, Vintage, New York, 1988

Parker, R., and Ganyon, J. (eds), *Conceiving Sexuality*, Routledge & Kegan Paul, New York, 1995

Pascal, M., *Varieties of Man/Boy Love: Modern Western Contexts*, Wallace Hamilton Press, New York, 1992

Pearsall, R., *The Worm in the Bud: The World of Victorian Sexuality*, Weidenfeld & Nicholson, London, 1969

Peck, J. R., and Feldman, M. W., 'Kin Selection and the Evolution of Monogamy', *Science*, 240:1672–4, 1988

Pennebaker, J. W., Dyer, M. A., *et al.*, 'Don't the Girls Get Prettier at Closing Time: A Country and Western Application to Psychology', *Personality and Social Psychology Bulletin*, 5:1, 122–5, 1979

Penzer, N. M., *The Harem*, Harrap, London, 1936

Perrett, D. I., and Benson, P., 'Face to Face With the Perfect Image', *New Scientist*, 22 February 1992

Perrett, D. I., May, K. A., and Yoshikawa, S., 'Facial Shape and Judgements of Female Attractiveness', *Nature*, 368:239–42

Phillips, R., *Putting Asunder: A History of Divorce in Western Society*, CUP, Cambridge, 1988

Plato (trs. W. Hamilton), *The Symposium*, Penguin, London, 1951

Polhemus, T., and Randall, H., *Rituals of Love: Sexual Experiments, Erotic Possibilities*, Picador, London, 1994

Pomeroy, S. B., *Goddesses, Whores, Wives and Slaves: Women in Classical Antiquity*, Schocken, New York, 1975

Porter, R., and Teich, M., *Sexual Knowledge, Sexual Science: The History of Attitudes to Sexuality*, CUP, Cambridge, 1994

Quale, G. R., *A History of Marriage Systems*, Greenwood Press, Westport (CT), 1988

Quinsey, V. L., and Lalumiere, M. L., 'Evolutionary Perspectives on Sexual Offending', *Sexual Abuse: A Journal of Research and Treatment*, 7:4, 301–15, 1995

Radway, J. A., *Reading the Romance*, Verso, London, 1987

Rattray Taylor, G., *Sex in History*, Ballantine, New York, 1954

Reid, R., 'Medical Aspects of Gender Identity Disorder (Transsexualism) and Their Legal Relevance', talk given at the Jubilee Rooms, House of Commons, London, 30 June 1994

Reinisch, J. R., and Beasley, R., *The Kinsey Institute New Report on Sex*, St Martin's Press, New York, 1990

Riddle, J. M., *Contraception and Abortion from the Ancient World to the Renaissance*, Harvard University Press, Cambridge (MA), 1994

Ridley, M., *Evolution*, Blackwell, Oxford, 1994

Ridley, M., *The Red Queen*, Viking, London, 1993

——, *The Origins of Virtue*, Viking, London, 1996

Rose, S., Lewontin, R. C., and Kamin, L. J., *Not In Our Genes: Biology, Ideology and Human Nature*, Pantheon, London, 1994

Rowland, D. A., and Perrett, D. I., 'Manipulating Facial Appearance through Shape and Colour', *Computer Graphics*, 70–6, September 1995

Rowland, D. L., Heiman, J. R., Gladue, B. A., *et al.*, 'Endocrine, Psychological and Genital Response to Sexual Arousal in Men', *Psychoneuroendocrinology*, 12:2, 149–58, 1987

Rubinow, D. R., and Schmidt, P. J., 'Androgens, Brain and Behavior', *American Journal of Psychiatry*, 153:8, 974–84, 1996

——, 'Psychoneuroendocrinology', in H. I. Kaplan and B. J. Sadock (eds), *Comprehensive Textbook of Psychiatry IV*, Williams & Wilkins, Baltimore, 1995

Rugoff, M., *Prudery and Passion: Sexuality in Victorian America*, Rupert Hart-Davis, London, 1972

Rusbridger, A., *A Concise History of the Sex Manual*, Faber & Faber, London, 1986

Ruse, M., *Homosexuality: A Philosophical Enquiry*, Blackwell, Oxford, 1988

Russett, C. E., *Sexual Science: The Victorian Construction of Womanhood*, Harvard University Press, Cambridge (MA), 1989

Sadalla, E. K., Kenrick, D. T., and Vershure, B., 'Dominance and Heterosexual Attraction', *Journal of Personality and Social Psychology*, 52:4, 730–8, 1987

Sanders, E. P., *The Historical Figure of Jesus*, Penguin, London, 1993

Scharff, D. E., *The Sexual Relationship: An Object Relations View of Sex and the Family*, Routledge & Kegan Paul, London, 1982

Scheib, J. A., 'Female Choice in the Context of Donor Insemination', in P. A. Gowaty (ed.), *Feminism and Evolutionary Biology: Boundaries, Intersections and Frontiers*, Chapman & Hall, New York, 1997

Shaw, B. D., 'Explaining Incest: Brother–Sister Marriage in Graeco-Roman Egypt' in *Man*, 27.2:267–99, 1992

Shepher, J., 'Mate Selection Among Second-generation Kibbutz Adolescents: Incest Avoidance and Negative Imprinting, *Archives of Sexual Behaviour*, I:293–307, 1971

——, *Incest: A Biosocial View*, Academic Press, New York, 1983

Sherfey, M. J., *The Nature and Evolution of Female Sexuality*, Vintage, New York, 1972

Short, R. V., and Balaban, E. (eds), *The Differences Between the Sexes*, CUP, Cambridge, 1994

Simon, W., *Postmodern Sexualities*, Routledge & Kegan Paul, London, 1996

Singh, D., 'Body Shapes and Women's Attractiveness: The Critical Role of Waist-Hip Ratio', *Human Nature*, 4:3, 297–321, 1993

——, 'Adaptive Significance of Female Physical Attractiveness: Role of Waist-to-hip Ratio', *Journal of Personality and Social Psychology*, 65:2, 293–307, 1993

Slob, A. K., Bax, C. M., Rowland, D. L., *et al.*, 'Sexual Arousability and the Menstrual Cycle', *Psychoneuroendocrinology*, 21:6, 545–58, 1996

Slob, A. K., Ernste, M., and van der Werff ten Bosch, J. J., 'Menstrual Cycle Phase and Sexual Arousability in Women', *Archives of Sexual Behavior*, 20:6, 567–77, 1991

Slob, A. K., and van der Werff ten Bosch, J. J., 'The Fundamental Role of Gonadal Steroids in Sexual Behaviour', *Balliere's Clinical Psychiatry*, 3:1, 1–24, 1997

Smith, E. R., Byrne, D., Becker, M. A., and Przybyla, D. P. J., 'Sexual Attitudes of Males and Females as Predictors of Interpersonal Attraction and Marital Compatibility', *Journal of Applied Social Psychology*, 23, 1011–34, 1993

Smith, J. R., and Smith, L. G., *Beyond Monogamy: Recent Studies of Sexual Alternatives in Marriage*, Johns Hopkins University Press, Baltimore, 1974

Smith, R. L. (ed.), *Sperm Competition and the Evolution of Animal Mating Systems*, Academic Press, Orlando, 1984

Solomon, R. C., *Love: Emotion, Myth and Metaphor*, Prometheus, Buffalo (NY), 1990

Spencer, C., *Homosexuality: A History*, Fourth Estate, London, 1995

Spiro, M. E., *Children of the Kibbutz*, Harvard University Press, Cambridge (MA), 1958

Sprenger, J., and Kramer, H. (trs. M. Summers), *Malleus Maleficarum*, John Rodker, London, 1928

Stearns, S. C. (ed.), *The Evolution of Sex and Its Consequences*, Binkhauser Press, Basel 1987

Steele, V., *Fetish: Fashion, Sex and Power*, OUP, Oxford, 1996

Stendhal, (trs. G. and S. Sale), *Love*, Penguin, London, 1975

Sternberg, R., and Barnes, M. (eds), *The Psychology of Love*, Yale University Press, New Haven, 1988

Stevens, A., and Price, J., *Evolutionary Psychiatry: A New Beginning*, Routledge & Kegan Paul, London, 1996

Stoddart, D. M., *The Scented Ape: The Biology and Culture of Human Odour*, CUP, Cambridge, 1990

Stone, L., *The Family, Sex and Marriage in England, 1500–1800*, Harper Torchbook, New York, 1979

——, 'Sex in the West', *The New Republic*, 8 July 1985

——, *The Past and the Present Revisited*, Routledge & Kegan Paul, London, 1987

——, *Road to Divorce: England, 1530–1987*, OUP, Oxford, 1990

——, *Uncertain Unions and Broken Lives*, OUP, Oxford, 1992

Stubrin, J. P., *Sexualities and Homosexualities*, Karnac, London, 1994

Swaab, D. F., 'Desirable biology', *Nature*, 382, 22 August 1996

Swaab, D. F., Gooren, L. J. G., and Hofman, M. A., 'The Human Hypothalamus in Relation to Gender and Sexual Orientation', *Progress in Brain Research*, 93:205–19, 1992

Swaab, D. F., and Hofman, M. A., 'Sexual Differentiation of the Human Hypothalamus: Ontogeny of the Sexually Dimorphic Nucleus of the Preoptic Area', *Developmental Brain Research*, 44, 314–18, 1988

——, 'An Enlarged Suprachiasmatic Nucleus in Homosexual Men', *Brain Research*, 537, 141–8, 1990

——, 'Sexual Differentiation of the Human Hypothalamus in Relation to Gender and Sexual Orientation', *TINS*, 18:6, 264–70, 1995

Swaab, D. F., Zhou, J. N., Fodor, M., and Hofman, M. A., 'Gender and Sexual Orientation-related Differences in the Human Hypothalamus', *Frontiers in Endocrinology*, 20, 135–52, 1996

Symons, D., *The Evolution of Human Sexuality*, OUP, New York, 1979

——, 'Precis of *The Evolution of Human Sexuality*', *Behavioural and Brain Sciences*, 3, 171–214, 1980

——, 'Another Woman That Never Existed', review of S. Hrdy's *The Woman That Never Evolved*, *The Quarterly Review of Biology*, 57:3, 297–300, 1982

——, 'Darwinism and Contemporary Marriage' in K. Davis (ed.), *Contemporary Marriage*, Russell Sage Foundation, New York, 1985

——, 'An Evolutionary Approach: Can Darwin's View of Life Shed Light on Human Sexuality?' in J. H. Geer and W. O'Donohue (eds), *Theories of Human Sexuality*, Plenum Press, New York, 1987

——, 'Beauty is in the Adaptations of the Beholder . . .' in P. R. Abramson and S. D. Pinkerton (eds), *Sexual Nature, Sexual Culture*, University of Chicago Press, Chicago, 1995

——, 'Neoteny Reconsidered', comment on Doug Jones' 'Sexual Selection, Physical Attractiveness and Facial Neoteny', *Current Anthropology*, 1996

Symons, D., and Ellis, B., 'Sex Differences in Sexual Fantasy: An Evolutionary Psychological Approach', *Journal of Sex Research*, 27: 527–55, 1990

——, 'Human Male-Female Differences in Sexual Desire' in A. E. Rasa, C. Vogel and E. Voland (eds), *The Sociobiology of Sexual and Reproductive Strategies*, Chapman & Hall, New York, 1989

Tannahill, R., *Sex in History*, Stein & Day, New York, 1980

Taylor, T., *The Prehistory of Sex*, Fourth Estate, London, 1996

Tennov, D., *Love and Limerence: The Experience of Being in Love*, Stein & Day, New York, 1979

Thompson, C. J. S., *Poisons and Poisoners*, Harold Shaylor, London, 1931

Thomson, O., *A History of Sin*, Canongate, Edinburgh, 1993

Thornhill, N. W., 'Characteristics of Female Desirability: Facultative Standards of Beauty', *Behavioural and Brain Sciences*, 12:35–6, 1989

——, 'The Evolutionary Significance of Incest Rules', *Ethology and Sociobiology*, 11: 113–29, 1989

Thornhill, N. W., and Thornhill, R., 'Human Rape: An Evolutionary Analysis', *Ethology and Sociobiology*, 4:137–73, 1983

——, 'The Evolutionary Psychology of Men's Coercive Sexuality', *Behavioural and Brain Sciences*, 15, 363–421, 1992

Thornhill, R., 'Is There Psychological Adaptation to Rape?', *Analyse and Kritik* 16, July 1994

Thornhill, R., and Bryant Furlow, F., 'The Orgasm Wars', *Psychology Today*, January-February 1996

Thornhill, R., and Gangestad, S., 'Human Facial Beauty: Averageness, Symmetry, and Parasite Resistance', *Human Nature*, 4:3, 237–69, 1993

——, 'Human Fluctuating Asymmetry and Sexual Behaviour', *Psychological Science*, 5:5, 297–302, 1994

——, 'The Evolution of Human Sexuality', *TREE*, 11:2, 98–102, 1996

Thornhill, R., Gangestad, S., and Comer, R., 'Human Female Orgasm and Mate Fluctuating Asymmetry', *Animal Behaviour*, 50, 1601–15, 1995

Thornhill, R., Gangestad, S., and Yeo, R., 'Facial Attractiveness, Developmental Stability and Fluctuating Asymmetry', *Ethology and Sociobiology*, 15:73–85, 1994

Thornhill, R., Pape Moller, A., and Soler, M., 'Breast Asymmetry, Sexual Selection and Human Reproductive Success', *Ethology and Sociobiology*, 16:207–19, 1995

Thornhill, R., and Watson, P., 'Fluctuating Asymmetry and Sexual Selection', *TREE*, 9:1, 21–5, 1994

Tiger, L., *The Pursuit of Pleasure*, Little, Brown, London, 1991

Tiger, L., and Robinson, M. H. (eds), *Man and Beast Revisited*, Smithsonian Institution, Washington DC, 1991

Tissot, S. A., *A Treatise on the Diseases Produced by Onanism. Translated from a New Edition of the French, with Notes and Appendix by an American Physician, New York, 1832*; facsimile reprint edition in C. Rosenberg and C. Smith-Rosenberg (eds), *The Secret Vice Exposed! Some Arguments Against Masturbation*, Arno Press, New York, 1974

Tooby, J., 'Pathogens, Polymorphism and the Evolution of Sex', *Journal of Theoretical Biology*, 97:557–76, 1982

——, 'The Emergence of Evolutionary Psychology' in D. Pines (ed.), *Emerging Syntheses in Science*, Santa Fe Institute, Santa Fe (NM), 1987

Tooby, J., and Cosmides, L., 'The Innate Versus the Manifest: How Universal Does a Universal Have to Be?', *Behavioural and Brain Sciences*, 12: 36–7, 1989

——, 'Adaptation Versus Phylogeny: The Role of Animal Psychology in the Study of Human Behavior', *International Journal of Comparative Psychology*, 2:3, 175–88, 1989

——, 'The Past Explains the Present: Emotional Adaptations and the Structure of Ancestral Environments', *Ethology and Sociobiology*, 11:375–424, 1990

——, 'On the Universality of Human Nature and the Uniqueness of the Individual: The Role of Genetics and Adaptation', *Journal of Personality*, 58:1, 17–67, 1990

——, 'The Psychological Foundations of Culture', in J. H. Barkow, J. Tooby and L. Cosmides (eds), *The Adapted Mind*, OUP, New York, 1992

Townsend, J. M., and Levy, G. D., 'Effects of Potential Partners' Physical Attractiveness and Socio-economic Status on Sexuality and Partner Selection', *Archives of Sexual Behaviour*, 311, 149–64, 1990

Travin, S., and Protter, B., *Sexual Perversion: Integrative Treatment Approaches for the Clinician*, Plenum Press, New York, 1993

Trivers, R. L., 'The Evolution of Reciprocal Altruism', *The Quarterly Review of Biology*, 46:35–7, 1971

——, 'Parental Investment and Sexual Selection' in B. Campbell (ed.), *Sexual Selection and the Descent of Man*, Aldine-Atherton, Chicago, 1972

——, 'Parent–Offspring Conflict', *American Zoologist*, 14:249–64, 1974

Tyldesley, J., *Daughters of Isis: Women of Ancient Egypt*, Penguin, London, 1994

Tysoe, M., *Love Isn't Quite Enough: The Psychology of Male–Female Relationships*, Fontana, London, 1992

Uvnas-Moberg, K., 'Breastfeeding: Physiological, Endocrine and Behavioural Adaptations Caused by Oxytocin and Local Neurogenic Activity in the Nipple and Mammary Gland', *Acta Paediatrica*, 1995

——, 'Physiological and Endocrine Effects of Social Contact', *Annals of the New York Academy of Science: Neurobiology of Affiliation*, 1995

——, 'Our Undiscovered "Peace and Calm" Hormones', *AMTA*, May 1996

——, 'Neuroendocrinology of the Mother–Child Interaction', *TEM*, 7:4, 1996

Valero, H., *Yanoáma: The Story of a Woman Abducted by Brazilian Indians*, Allen & Unwin, London, 1969

van den Berghe, P. L., *Human Family Systems: An Evolutionary View*, Greenwood Press, Westport (CT), 1979

van den Berghe, P. L., and Mesher, G. M., 'Royal Incest and Inclusive Fitness', *American Ethnologist*, 7.2.300–17, 1980 van den Berghe, P. L., and Frost, P., 'Skin Colour Preference, Sexual Dimorphism and Sexual Selection: A Case of Gene Culture Co-evolution?', *Ethnic and Racial Studies*, 9: 87–113, 1986

van Gulik, R., *Sexual Life in Ancient China: A Preliminary Survey of Chinese Sex and Society from c. 1500 BC until AD 1644*, E. J. Brill, Leiden, 1974

Vatsyayana (trs. Sir Richard Burton and F. F. Arbuthnot), *Kama Sutra*, Luxor Press, London, 1963

Walker Bynum, C., *Holy Feast and Holy Fast: The Religious Significance of Food to Medieval Women*, University of California Press, Los Angeles, 1987

——, *Fragmentation and Redemption: Essays on Gender and the Human Body in Medieval Religion*, Urzone Publishers, New York, 1991

——, *The Resurrection of the Body in Western Christianity, 200–1336*, Columbia University Press, New York, 1995

Wallen, K., 'Desire and Ability: Hormones and the Regulation of Female Sexual Behaviour', *Neuroscience and Behavioural Reviews*, 14:233–41, 1990

——, 'The Evolution of Female Sexual Desire', in P. Abramson and S. Pinkerton (eds), *Sexual Nature, Sexual Culture*, University of Chicago Press, Chicago, 1995

Waller, N. G. and Shaver, P. R., 'The Importance of Nongenetic Influences on Romantic Love Styles: A Twin-Family Study', *Psychological Science*, 5:5, 268–74, 1994

Walsh, A., *The Science of Love: Understanding Love and Its Effects on Mind and Body*, Prometheus, Buffalo (NY), 1991

Walsh, H., *Mandatory Celibacy and Sexual Ethics in the Latin Rite of the Roman Catholic Church*, D. Ed dissertation manuscript, 1994

——, *Bowsie* (manuscript)

Walster, E., and Walster, G. W., 'Effect of Expecting to be Liked on Choice of Associates', *Journal of Personality and Social Psychology*, 67, 402–4, 1963

Warner, Marina, *Alone of All Her Sex: The Myth and Cult of the Virgin Mary*, Picador, London, 1990

Webb, Peter, *The Erotic Arts*, New York Graphics Society, Boston, 1975

Wedekind, C., Seebeck, T., Bettens, F., and Paepke, A. J., 'MHC-dependent Mate Preferences in Humans', *Proceedings of the Royal Society of London*, B 260, 245–9, 1995

Weeks, J., *Sexuality*, Routledge & Kegan Paul, New York, 1986

Weinberg, T. S., *S&M: Strategies in Dominance and Submission*, Prometheus, Buffalo (NY), 1995

Weinrich, J. D., *Sexual Landscapes*, Scribner, New York, 1987

Welldon, Estela V., *Mother, Madonna, Whore*, The Guilford Press, London, 1988

——, 'Women As Abusers', in K. Abel, M. Buscewicz *et al.* (eds), *Planning Community Mental Health Services for Women*, Routledge, London, n.d.

——, 'Female Perversion and the Hollywood Touch' (no date or publication details)

——, 'Equality is not Sameness: A Psychoanalytic View of the Sexes', *Indian Journal of Social Work*, LIII:3, 429, 1992

——, 'Female Sex Offenders', *Prison Service Journal*, 107, 39–47, 1996

——, 'Perversions in Men and Women', *British Journal of Psychotherapy*, 12:4, 480–6, 1996

Wellings, K., Field, J., Johnson, A. M., and Wadsworth, J., *Sexual Behaviour in Britain: the National Survey of Sexual Attitudes and Lifestyles*, Penguin, London, 1994

Westermarck, E., *The History of Human Marriage* (5th edn), Allerton Press, New York, 1922

Westphal, K., 'Die kontrare Sexualempfindung: Symptom eines neuropathologischen (psychopathischen) Zustandes', *Archiv für Psychiatrie und Nervenkrankeiten*, 2:73–108, 1869

Whitehurst, R. N., 'Violence Potential in Extramarital Sexual Responses', *Journal of Marriage and the Family*, 33: 683–91

Wiederman, M. W., 'Evolved Gender Differences in Mate Preferences: Evidence from Personal Advertisements', *Ethology and Sociobiology*, 14:331–52, 1993

——, 'Women, Sex and Food: A Review of Research on Eating Disorders and Sexuality', *Journal of Sex Research*, 33:4, 301–11, 1996

Wiederman, M. W., and Allgeier, E. R., 'Gender Differences in Sexual Jealousy: Adaptationist or Social Learning Explanation?', *Ethology and Sociobiology*, 14:115–40, 1993

Williams, G. C., *Adaptation and Natural Selection: A Critique of Some Current Evolutionary Thought*, Princeton University Press, Princeton, 1974

——, *Sex and Evolution*, Princeton University Press, Princeton, 1975

——, *Plan and Purpose in Nature*, HarperCollins, New York, 1997

Williams, L., *Hard Core*, Pandora, London, 1990

Wilson, A. N., *Jesus*, HarperCollins, London, 1993

Wilson, E. O., *Sociobiology: The New Synthesis*, Harvard University Press, Cambridge (MA), 1975

——, *On Human Nature*, Harvard University Press, Cambridge (MA), 1978

Wilson, G. D., 'The Psychology of Male Sexual Arousal', in A. Gregoire and J. P. Prior (eds), *Impotence: An Integrated Approach to Clinical Practice*, Churchill Livingstone, Edinburgh, 1993

——, 'Gender Differences in Sexual Fantasy: An Evolutionary Analysis', *Person. Individ. Differences*, 22:1, 27–31, 1997

Wilson, G. D., and Barrett, P. T., 'Parental Characteristic and Partner Choice: Some Evidence for Oedipal Imprinting', *Journal of Biosocial Sciences*, 19:157–61, 1987

Wilson, M., and Daly, M., 'The Man Who Mistook His Wife for a Chattel', in J. H. Barkow, L. Cosmides and J. Tooby (eds), *The Adapted Mind*, OUP, New York, 1992

——, 'Spousal Homicide Risk and Estrangement', *Violence and Victims*, 8:1, 3–1993

——, 'Who Kills Whom in Spouse Killings? On the Exceptional Sex Ratio of Spousal Homicides in the United States', *Criminology*, 30:2, 189–215, 1992

Wilson, M., Daly, M., Dobash, R. P., and Dobash, R. E., 'The Myth of Sexual Symmetry in Marital Violence', *Social Problems*, 39:1, 71–91, 1992

Wilson, M., Daly, M., and Johnson, H., 'Lethal and Non-lethal Violence Against Wives', *Canadian Journal of Criminology*, 37:331–61, 1995

Wilson, M., Daly, M., and Singh, L., 'Children Fathered by Previous Partners: A Risk Factor for Violence Against Women', *Canadian Journal of Public Health*, 84:209–10, 1993

Wright, R., *The Moral Animal: Why We Are the Way We Are*, Little, Brown, London, 1995

Zhou, J. N., Hofman, M. A., Gooren, L., and Swaab, D. F., 'A Sex Difference in the Human Brain and Its Relation to Transsexuality', *Nature*, 378, 68–70

Zhou, J. N., Hofman, M. A., and Swaab, D. F., 'No Changes in the Number of Vasoactive Intestinal Polypeptide-expressing Neurons in the Suprachiasmatic Nucleus of Homosexual Men; Comparison With Vasopressin-Expressing Neurons', *Brain Research*, 672, 285–8, 1995

Index

Abacus now offers an exciting range of quality titles by both established and new authors. All of the books in this series are available from:

Little, Brown and Company (UK),
P.O. Box 11,
Falmouth,
Cornwall TR10 9EN.

Fax No: 01326 317444.
Telephone No: 01326 372400
E-mail: books@barni.avel.co.uk

Payments can be made as follows: cheque, postal order (payable to Little, Brown and Company) or by credit cards, Visa/Access. Do not send cash or currency. UK customers and B.F.P.O. please allow £1.00 for postage and packing for the first book, plus 50p for the second book, plus 30p for each additional book up to a maximum charge of £3.00 (7 books plus).

Overseas customers including Ireland, please allow £2.00 for the first book plus £1.00 for the second book, plus 50p for each additional book.

NAME (Block Letters) ....

....

ADDRESS ....

....

....

☐ I enclose my remittance for ....

☐ I wish to pay by Access/Visa Card

Number ☐☐☐☐☐☐☐☐☐☐☐☐☐☐☐☐☐

Card Expiry Date ☐☐☐☐